Curriculum Revolution: Mandate For Change

Pub. No. 15-2224

National League for Nursing

ISBN 0-88737-404-2

The views expressed in this publication represent the views of the authors and do not necessarily reflect the official views of the National League for Nursing.

Second printing 1.5M-0491-029950
Printed in the United States of America

Contents

Contributors

Mila Ann Aroskar, EdD, RN, FAAN, is Associate Professor, School of Public Health, University of Minnesota, Minneapolis, Minnesota.

Em Olivia Bevis, MA, RN, FAAN, is Nursing Educational Consultant, Bluffon, South Carolina, and Adjunct Professor of Research, Georgia Southern College, Statesboro, Georgia.

Carolyn Oiler Boyd, EdD, RN, is Associate Professor, College of Nursing, Villanova University, Villanova, Pennsylvania.

Sheila A. Corcoran, PhD, RN, is Associate Professor, School of Nursing, University of Minnesota, Minneapolis, Minnesota.

Susan E. Costello, DNSc, RN, is Director of Nursing Education and Research, Georgetown University Hospital, Washington, DC.

Nancy Diekelmann, PhD, RN, FAAN, is Professor, School of Nursing, University of Wisconsin, Madison, Wisconsin.

Nancy P. Greenleaf, DNSc, RN, is Dean, University of Southern Maine, Portland, Maine.

Lucille A. Joel, EdD, RN, FAAN, is Chairperson, Department of Adults and the Aged, College of Nursing, Rutgers, The State University of New Jersey, Newark, New Jersey.

Carol Lindeman, PhD, RN, FAAN, is Dean, School of Nursing, Oregon Health Sciences University, Portland, Oregon.

Patricia Moccia, PhD, RN, is Chairperson, Department of Nursing

Education, Teachers College, Columbia University, New York, New York.

Patricia L. Munhall, EdD, RN, is Professor, Hunter-Bellevue School of Nursing, Hunter College of the City University of New York, New York, New York.

Christine Tanner, PhD, RN, FAAN, is Professor and Director, Office of Research Development and Utilization, School of Nursing, Oregon Health Sciences University, Portland, Oregon.

Theresa M. Valiga, EdD, RN, is Associate Professor, College of Nursing, Villanova University, Villanova, Pennsylvania.

Jean Watson, PhD, RN, FAAN, is Dean and Professor, School of Nursing, University of Colorado Health Sciences Center, Denver, Colorado.

Alma S. Woolley, EdD, RN, is Dean, Georgetown University School of Nursing, Washington, DC.

Preface

As nursing moves into the last decade of the 20th century, nursing educators continue to focus ever more critically on the nursing curriculum. To transform the nursing curriculum will mean a transformation in nurses themselves, and thus of nursing. What is at stake, and which appears as a common theme in the papers presented, is the human aspect of nursing, and a broadening and enhancing of educational perspectives that speak to that theme. Rather than relying on older models of curriculum development which, to a large degree, are structured on *training* rather than *education*, on *technique* rather than *understanding*, the authors prefer new, multifaceted, and more philosophical models that build on past successes but reject their shortcomings. Whether the subject is DRGs; the effect of fee-for-service medicine on both patient and nurse; changing patterns in the nursing labor force; research in undergraduate curriculum; innovations in clinical teaching; research in clinical judgment; cognitive development; or phenomenology as a philosophical perspective particularly relevant to the analysis of caring, a singular recognition presides: Current models of nursing curriculum development are in dire need of revision or outright rejection.

The radical character of this recognition is both animating and cautionary. The nurse educators presented in this volume clearly recognize the difficulties of the struggle before them. Now that sufficient time has passed since nursing achieved its goal of academic recognition, it must accomplish something more. It must, in analyzing itself, understand and capitalize on its essential function, which is and has always been *caring*.

Nursing must come to understand caring as it never has before. Indeed, it must re-create its curriculum around it. Rather than continue to use current models of learning and structure nursing curriculum around standard evaluation instruments alone, or be an even "unwilling" partner to economic and social policies that consider wellness as the result of specific medical procedures rather than as a holistic quality of life itself, nursing must respond, and it must respond critically and intelligently. It must look to new perspectives to deal with the inadequacies of its present curriculum models as it faces an ever challenging future.

The papers presented here speak to such pressing topics and more. Initially presented at the National League for Nursing's Fourth Conference on Nursing Education in 1987, they have been published with the aim of sharing the enthusiasms, alternative strategies, criticisms, and concerns of the speakers to nurses and nurse educators nationwide.

1

A Case Study: Curriculum in Transition

Jean Watson

HUMAN CARING AS MORAL CONTEXT FOR NURSING EDUCATION

In the midst of all the debate about the future of nursing education, it is clear that nursing education has historically failed in two significant ways. First, we educators have failed to address the issue of how to educate a person and have continued to prepare a first-level "product" for institutions. Second, we have failed to address the issue of how to prepare educated nurses as full health care giving professionals and have focused instead on how to prepare students to be institutional employees (Watson, 1987).

Because of our failure to address these issues, the overall goals of nursing education have become inverted. Nursing has adopted a rationalist-objectivist model of education as well as an objectivist model of medical science—which means, essentially, that it has come to neglect the philosophical, moral context of health and human caring. Now, at last, we are beginning to realize that nursing education must attend to education of the whole person and recognize that learning is subjective, contextual, dialogic, and values-driven. We are beginning to acknowledge the conflicts that exist between our theories of education and our curricular practices; between our philosophies, theories, and beliefs about health and human caring and our professional nursing practices; and between our educational programs, with all the scientific-technical knowledge they contain, and our expectations for professional clinical care. We are beginning to recognize that one can have an extensive command of scientific facts and theories and be technically an expert without being be a true professional. In the new vision we are developing, professional education must also include exposure to liberal arts, encouragement of critical thinking, and a moral context for advanced professional education that is based upon a contextual human science educational model.

We need to establish a moral context for the new liberal nursing education we envision. It is becoming increasingly clear that health and human caring processes in nursing require a special way of being. We can be technically and scientifically correct but still make moral or normative errors. More and more, it seems that what is needed is subordination of knowledge, meaning, and technique to morals and a way of being as a caring professional—in other words, a shift from doing to being, a shift to new epistemologies, new ontologies, and new teaching-learning methodologies. The urgency of such a shift becomes especially great in light of the recent literature on increasing specialization and the objectivist model of nursing curricula.

One argument for the precedence of the moral context over the technical context is that this precedence is a true reflection of the nature of the professional-client relationship itself. In this view, caring is the moral ideal that guides the nurse through the caregiving process, and knowledgeable caring (i.e., professional nursing) is the highest form of commitment, an end in and of itself.

Thus, the moral context for nursing education as health and human caring becomes associated with a professional way of being, which raises serious questions for schools of nursing. Schools will have to reconsider many of the things they have traditionally done, such as

- treating students as objects;
- using mechanical or industrial terms, such as "products" and "aggregates";
- focusing on cognitive-technical outcomes alone, thereby creating competency without compassion or caring;
- restricting teaching-learning to behavioral objectives, factual information, and techniques;
- tolerating power and dependence roles for teachers and learners;
- separating doing from knowing and from being;
- tolerating accreditation processes that are in direct conflict with nursing's moral and scientific beliefs and educational philosophies and theories; and

- fixating on entry into practice and a degree rather than how to educate thinking professional people in such a way as to prepare them for a full health and human caring role that is consistent with nursing's social, moral, and scientific mission to society.

Our emerging new consciousness is issuing a call for new actions, for a revolution. We must have the courage to give up what is antiquated and no longer works.

@ the same time we must not throw out what works

CREATING A NEW PROFESSIONAL NURSE

As part of the moral-social action initiatives in Colorado, the University of Colorado School of Nursing is engaged in research aimed at contributing to the development of a new health and human caring science model and a new educational model for preparing professional nurses. The moral context of health and human caring in nursing within a humanitarian paradigm is the starting point and is guiding the School in its research. All of us at the School are motivated by nursing's duty to be accountable to society for health; by its caring and healing ideals; by its knowledge, values, and technologies; and by its caring expertise.

Curricula in Transition

In an effort to make the shift I spoke of earlier, we at the University of Colorado have decided to

- acknowledge and act on caring as a moral ideal and incorporate philosophical theories of human caring, health, and healing into our curricula;
- acknowledge and act on our commitment to prepare nurses as both educated persons and full health and human caring professionals.
- acknowledge the arts and humanities as essential for educated persons and caring professionals;
- include aspects of health, healing, and human caring knowledge and practices that are not yet generally considered part of the standard nursing curricula;
- adopt a humanitarian paradigm that identifies the humanities, social-biomedical science, and human caring content and process as the core of scholarly academic activities and clinical care practices;

- adopt a contextual approach in teaching the subjective, philosophical, and ethical/caring responsibilities of nurses as full health professionals.
- acknowledge faculty development needs for new teaching-learning methods and student-teacher interactive practices—e.g., shift from oppressive interactions to liberating interactions (or from maintenance learning to anticipatory-participatory learning) or emphasize faculty's role as expert learners rather than expert givers of information (Botkin, Elmandra, & Malitza, 1984);
- foster faculty and student creativity in finding new and different approaches to in-depth study of concepts of caring in human health and healing, perhaps including development of courses using art, music, literature, poetry, drama, and movement as means of examining subjective responses to health and illness, as well as examination of new caring-healing modalities; and
- restructure practice roles by piloting new professional practice roles and new kinds of clinical colleagues in traditional and nontraditional health care delivery systems.

In so deciding, the School is publicly acknowledging that Humpty-Dumpty has fallen, and the pieces cannot be put back together. We believe that today the nursing profession is being challenged to create a new, professional nurse who is a full health and human caring professional, or else to become obsolete.

THE NURSE DOCTORATE IN HUMAN CARING, HEALTH, AND HEALING

In our view, the preferred future for nursing education is a post-baccalaureate program in human caring, health, and healing that leads to the nursing doctorate (ND) degree. The following are the proposed components of the educational base of this program (Watson, 1988, p. 43):

- a more extensive liberal arts foundation that focuses on understanding of and appreciation for cultural diversity and on the human subjective dimensions of health-illness experiences;
- training in critical thinking and advanced problem solving, contributing to clinical judgments and independent decision making;

- a core knowledge underpinning of biomedical science, social behavioral science, and organization/system management theory and practice;
- a more extensive training in philosophical and ethical decision-making skills that is based on ethics of human caring, which addresses contextual, compassionate, relational, ethical dilemmas, as well as on the traditional rationalistic approach to principle-based biomedical ethics.
- exploration of the contextual value-laden relationship theory that is associated with human caring transactions, emphasizing self-care and more autonomous decision-making processes as important client goals in health care;
- a human caring theory-based nursing curriculum that takes into account the latest research into human caring practices and systems of caring and emphasizes the relationship between human and system caring approaches and health/healing outcomes (regardless of medical diagnosis and treatment regimen).

The following are the major desired outcomes of the ND program (Watson, 1988, p. 44):

- Graduates will have mastered both primary and tertiary practitioner skills, including physical and psychosocial assessment and management skills, especially in relation to elderly clients, chronically ill clients, children and adolescents, and developing families. They acquire and verify their skills within the context of human caring values, ethics, and the clinical knowledge base.
- Graduates will have familiarized themselves with new human caring practice modalities that incorporate natural healing approaches (along with traditional medical regimens) and esthetics-based approaches, such as music and movement therapy. These new modalities might also make use of other health-healing approaches that complement and balance traditional medical approaches, including stress management, therapeutic touch, imagery, expressive journaling, therapeutic massage, advanced interpersonal communication, and health teaching-learning skills.
- Graduates will have had access to a wide range of options with respect to both supportive-elective course work and clinical practice. They will have had experience in areas such as administrative management and clinical education, as well as in specific areas of clini-

cal practice such as acute or progressive life-threatening illness and health and wellness self-care.

Essentially, ND-prepared nurses will have discarded the non-nursing functions, tasks, and responsibilities that can be performed efficiently by others and consequently will function solely as expert caring clinicians. They will, however, retain the crucial human caring knowledge and practices considered to be the best of current nursing practice (Smith, 1987). Thus, ND-prepared nurses will be trained as full health and human caring professionals who are capable of making independent and critical clinical judgments. They will function as advanced nurse clinicians in institutions, homes, clinics, and alternative care settings. They will be capable of assessing and managing the care of patients or families with health-related needs, chronic illness-related needs, aging-associated needs, or acute tertiary health care needs. Their unique preparation and position will enable them to follow individuals and groups of patients on a continuing basis, in and out of hospitals and other systems, as well as to provide, oversee, or coordinate direct continuous care for people in society.

The ND in Society

In society, ND-prepared nurses will interact with other health professionals on an equal footing as acknowledged experts in health and human caring. Their last year of study and practice will be in a given setting or with a given population or age group. In this way, they can time the attainment of a certification option in a given specialty area of practice toward the end of study to coincide with a clinical internship.

The development of the ND program rests on several assumptions:

- The health care delivery system of the future will be a multifaceted, complex system of choices, both in traditional and nontraditional settings.
- Hospitals will continue to decline and eventually will accommodate only the most severely and acutely ill.
- Home care, family-oriented care, and self-care will continue to increase as people become better informed, more responsible, and more assertive with respect to their own health care needs.

The role of a full health professional nurse in and out of institutions —namely, to deliver expert caring and provide, oversee, or coordinate advanced health-healing practices—is one that will continue to be critical in the society of the future. Indeed, some futurists suggest that the expert caring nurse as full health professional will be the *only* continuous care provider in the largely depersonalized, technologically oriented, fragmented system of care that our current system is rapidly evolving into (Watson, 1988; Miller, 1984).

CONCLUSIONS

Eventually, ND-prepared nurses, as full health caring professionals, can help to bring about a new social order in the traditional health care delivery system and open up new continuous care options for health care in society. These professionals might fill a large void in the traditional, medically dominated, illness-focused health care system (Watson, 1988, p. 45).

REFERENCES

Botkin, J. W., Elmandra, M., & Malitza, M. (1984). *No limits to learning, bridging the human gap.* New York: Pergamon Press.

Miller, V. (1984). Nirvana in the year 2000. In J. Bilitski & M. Taylor (Eds.), *Nursing in the year 2000.* Morgantown, WV: West Virginia University Press.

Smith, A. (1987). Personal communication re: N.D. University of Colorado, School of Nursing.

Watson, J. (1987). The dream curriculum. In *Patterns on nursing: Strategic planning for nursing education.* New York: National League for Nursing.

Watson, J. (1988). The professional doctorate as an entry level into practice. In *NLN Perspectives.* New York: National League for Nursing.

BIBLIOGRAPHY

American Association of Colleges of Nursing. (1986). *Essentials of college and university education for professional nursing.* Washington, DC: Author.

Fry, S. (1988). The ethic of caring: Can it survive in nursing? *Nursing Outlook, 36*(1), 48.

Moccia, P. (1988). At the faultline: Social activism and caring. *Nursing Outlook, 36*(1), 30–33.

Sakalys, J. A., & Watson, M. J. (1985, September–October). New directions on higher education: A review of trends. *Journal of Professional Nursing,* pp. 293–299.

Sakalys, J. A., & Watson, M. J. (1986, March–April). Professional education: Postbaccalaureate education for professional nursing. *Journal of Professional Nursing*, pp. 91–97.

Schon, D. (1987). *Educating the reflective practitioner*. San Francisco: Jossey-Bass.

Special Supplement: Nurses for the future. (1988). *American Journal of Nursing, 87*(12), 1593–1657.

Tate, J. (1988). ND task group curricular materials. Unpublished manuscript, University of Colorado School of Nursing.

2

The Impact of DRGs on Basic Nursing Education and Curriculum Implications

Lucille A. Joel

ADVENT OF DRGs

Diagnosis-related groups (DRGs) are both a symbol of growing cost containment in health care and a milestone event in the movement towards greater economic control. Successful employment of DRGs hinges on a reshaping of the diagnostic and therapeutic management practices of physicians accomplished by restricting reimbursement to hospitals. Hospitals were originally targeted for change as the most costly component of the delivery system, and DRGs were proposed as a way of ensuring that government and the health care industry would share the risk of providing hospital services to Medicare recipients and that acute care resources would be allocated equitably to those who needed them most. The model promised rewards for efficient service delivery. Many hospitals, however, saw DRGs as offering more risk than reward and considered them a negative approach to cost control. More positive techniques for reshaping utilization practices have come from business and industry in the form of rewards to employees for acting as prudent consumers of health care. This difference in ap-

 This paper was supported under contract with Mid-Atlantic Regional Nursing Association.

proach between public and private-sector strategies is important: appeals to the provider and negative reinforcement can be usefully contrasted with appeals to the consumer and positive reinforcement.

A new mosaic of reimbursement practices has increased the acuity of hospital patients and created unrelenting pressure to decrease the length of stay and increase the volume of admissions. "High technology" has moved into home health care and nursing homes, since these offer less costly settings for care. Managed care systems and ambulatory services are beginning to dominate health care, and in so doing create a critical need for case management. Delivering care is no more important than developing independence and self-sufficiency in the client and mobilizing informal resources. The growing numbers of frail elderly persons and chronically ill patients in the population pose a challenge to the traditional medical ethic, as improvement in functional ability becomes as important as or more important than cure.

Even these few observations build an incontestable case for more and better prepared nurses. Too much is being expected of too few. The wide range of consumer need is creating a market for a sophisticated corps of professionals and associates who work under their direction but are not interchangeable with them. Educational programs for entry into practice should reflect distinctions between categories of nurses and should manifest substantial differences from pre-DRG programs.

An absence of change is cause for concern and raises the question of how well nursing is responding to current realities. In this regard, the findings of a recent survey of schools of nursing in states in the jurisdiction of the Mid-Atlantic Regional Nursing Association (MARNA, 1987) are discouraging. Only 52 percent of respondents claimed to have made any curriculum adaptations in response to DRGs. All the respondents agreed that there was an observable increase in patient acuity, but 55 percent saw no need for adjustments in clinical learning. Respondents generally described an increased emphasis on discharge planning, patient teaching (most noticeably in associate degree programs), and quality assurance. With disturbing honesty, 72 percent of the responding schools reported making no changes in their programs to bring their faculty up to date on the changing practice environment. Overall, respondents were concerned with the acuity of hospital experiences and the rapid turnover and decreasing numbers of hospital patients.

Though only 29 schools responded, I believe that the conclusion suggested by the data is essentially correct: nursing education is not responding adequately to the challenge of the times. This being the case, it is not surprising that graduates are disillusioned by contemporary practice and ill-equipped to respond to consumers' need for more sophisticated service.

In the remainder of this paper, I will detail the changing practice environment and its implications for curriculum in more detail. Where the experiences of MARNA states differ from those of the nation as a whole, I will say so. Much of the direction for change proposed in this paper is based on data and experience from the state of New Jersey, which was the setting for the initial experiments with the DRG system. These proposals for change are not futuristic: the future is now. Talk of "the future" creates a safe distance, and there is nothing safe about substituting rhetoric for action. The direction of change formalized in the DRG system has been evident for at least a decade. The persistence of inaction and comfort with traditional ways requires immediate attention if the potential damage is to be controlled. As we face the need for change, we should resist the temptation to try to prove the value of nurses and nursing. It is not necessary: we already have enough proof and consumer support to be able to proceed without apology.

NURSING AND THE CHANGING HEALTH CARE SYSTEM

The health professions grew out of social need. Their future depends on their ability to walk the fine line between acting in the best interests of the consumer and responding to changing times. As a class, the health professionals address a very distinct cluster of human concerns. These fields of work are characterized by "soft boundaries"; that is, over time activities may be transferred from one provider to another or become the common property of several provider professionals simultaneously. The health care system has experienced dramatic changes as a result of appropriate concern over the cost, quality, and availability of services. It is logical to assume that the health care professions will be expected to adjust their roles accordingly.

Governmental concern with the cost of health care began to surface shortly after the establishment of the Medicare and Medicaid programs. Simultaneously, private-sector health insurance became available to a growing number of citizens as a fringe benefit obtained through the workplace. Americans began to expect first-dollar comprehensive coverage from both public and private-sector insurers. Little effort was spent on trying to stem the tide of escalating health care cost until the accession of a federal administration that placed greater value on defense than on social welfare programs. Hospital expenses reimbursed under part A of Medicare were quickly targeted for cost control as the most expensive aspect of the one program fully under the federal government's control. Cost predictions for hospital management of medical and surgical conditions were developed through the merging of data on the prescriptive practices of physicians for Medicare recipients with the Diagnosis-Related Groups Classification System. The result was the much publicized DRG system, or, more correctly, the Medicare prospective pricing methodology based on case mix with episode of illness reimbursement. With the institution of this system, the government had set in motion a process that would totally transform the American health care delivery system (Joel, 1985).

Controls developed by the federal government for the Medicare system were quickly taken up by state Medicaid programs and private-sector insurers. Business and industry expanded the theme of cost-efficiency and began to insure their employees themselves instead of contracting with the insurance industry. This now common practice has created a private-sector environment that rewards self-care and prudent buyer practices and derives tangible benefit from investment in health (Joel, 1985). An observer might conclude that the private sector, fearing eventual government intrusion aimed at controlling escalating health care costs, found more creative approaches that will ultimately reshape the delivery system to a greater extent and in a more radical manner than DRGs have.

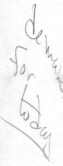

The roles and responsibilities of providers will have to be reassessed to complement a practice environment that is economically driven. The watchwords for today are self-care, home- and community-based services, case coordination and integration of services, information management, high technology, client advocacy, and personal accountability for care. Within a health care delivery system ensnared in complex calculations and regulations, there exists the expectation that operations will be fine-tuned to avoid waste and the assumption that only the most cost-efficient providers, settings, and services are justified.

Nurses have always been the most visible providers in the delivery system. Nurses have traditionally coordinated and integrated the treatment regimen, acted as patient advocates, and counseled and taught with the goal of returning the recipient of care to self-sufficiency and independence. As Lang (1987) puts it, "the nurse has created order out of chaos and health out of illness. . . . Nurses hold patients' dignity in their hands more often than their lives. . . . Nurses have come to view peaceful death as a therapeutic triumph."

The restructuring of the health care delivery system creates a temporary window of opportunity for these historical strengths of nursing. Should nurses hesitate, new providers may be created. For example, society created the physician's assistant in a time of physician undersupply, and it created the licensed practical nurse as a response to a nurse shortage. Alternatively, other providers may expand their boundaries to fill the breach. This is already happening, in fact. Social workers are functioning as case managers and discharge planners. Health educators intrude on the comprehensive care that characterizes nursing. Bioengineers, by virtue of their control of high technology, stand between nurses and their patients. Physicians, as their own surplus grows, begin to encroach on the practice of nursing; it is quite possible that very soon salaried physicians will be proposed as a remedy to the shortage of critical care nurses. History will repeat itself. Earlier in this century, when there was a physician shortage, nurses expanded their practice to include physical examinations, immunization, and additional well-child activities. These activities were reclaimed by physicians as their numbers increased (DeMaio, 1979).

NURSING'S HIGHLY INTERACTIVE TRADITION

Reimbursement models are creating a highly interactive future for health care. There is a trend toward capitated financing and managed care systems that will eventually limit both community and institutional resources, and toward increased acuity on the part of consumers in the health care delivery system. Fragmentation and complexity will post a constant threat to continuity and comprehensive care. Case coordination and service integration will cut costs and become desirable, if not essential. Nurses would be perfectly suited for such an interactive future, but so far nurses have not claimed an active role within it. In public programs such as long-term home care, in which case coordinator positions exist, regulations allow either social workers or nurses to occupy these positions.

The business literature presents case coordination as a significant enhancement to cost-efficiency. Industry reports a $3.00/employee return on a $1.00/employee investment into a combination of case coordination and utilization review. (Naisbitt & Aburdene, 1985). In other instances, comparable services have yielded an overall reduction of 20 percent in medical claims cost (Rutigliano, 1985). Such programs have provided for pre-certification of reimbursement limits, employee counseling about options in clinical management, advocacy in dealings with provider professionals (if the employee expresses the need), and analysis and policy development in high-volume claims areas. In one audit of employee claims for nonsurgical hospital treatment of lower back pain, 85 percent of inpatient days were determined to be inappropriate (Rutigliano, 1985). An expert panel concluded that the prevailing prescription of bed rest and medication could be provided more cheaply and safely at home with appropriate home-care support. Policies were subsequently revised to reflect new reimbursement parameters. The marriage of sophisticated clinical judgment and reimbursement policy is particularly significant in this case, because medical treatment of lower back pain is an exceptionally high-volume DRG. In New Jersey, for example, it is the most frequent DRG (New Jersey Department of Health, 1984).

Maximizing an individual's personal resources is no less challenging than integrating the health care system in their behalf. In the future, rewards will be offered for self-care and the supplementary use of services provided by friends, family, and volunteers. It is only logical that care should be given most painstakingly by those who care. Provider professionals who can develop resources that do not add to the cost of the system, that eliminate duplication, and that reshape consumer utilization practices will move into controlling positions. Advocacy will be visible to and valued by the consumer, who in fact has become the most significant player in the health care game. The role components I have been discussing—human resource development, coordination, and advocacy—are among the services nurses have historically provided. If to some extent they have slipped from our grasp, we must reclaim them.

Any contemplated alterations of our nursing curricula must reflect a renewed appreciation of the psychosocial and interactive aspects of practice, which have traditionally been extremely important in nursing. Nursing is the most interactive discipline in a highly interactive environment. This quality derives from the intimate and holistic nature of the service. The unique nurse-client relationship should be dignified in the curriculum through the development of a practice framework that promotes nursing as relevant to the times. The nurse complements the clients' deficits in self-care, with the aim of providing resources in the manner that clients would select for themselves, and always with an eye to promoting self-sufficiency and independence. Today, this philosophy is highly marketable, since it contributes to cost-efficiency. To build on this point, we must accord a higher priority to discharge planning and to teaching and counseling as therapeutic techniques for developing self-sufficiency.

The ability to establish excellent interdisciplinary relations is another guaranteed route to cost savings that is highly dependent on skilled interaction. Strong practice credibility and the capacity to function as part of a team are prerequisites for acquisition of this ability. Consumers have become intolerant of turf disputes between provider professionals—rightly so, since the net effect of these disputes is to divert energy from the mission of health care delivery. The nature of health professions demands that territorial boundaries between areas of practice remain flexible. Time and social necessity require a periodic rearangement of activity areas between disciplines. Tolerance for ambiguity and flexibility and impatience with vested interests serve consumers' interest best.

Interdisciplinary experiences are already a required component of nursing education programs, but in the years to come they should be given more serious attention than they have yet received. The ideal route to interdisciplinary respect and understanding is shared educational experience. In the best of all worlds, nursing education would include a health science core and a clinical laboratory that would allow students from a variety of disciplines to interact and provide care jointly. In this less than ideal world, educators should at least search out practice settings for students that allow participation in a multidisciplinary team.

Rutgers College of Nursing created such a learning situation in its Teaching Nursing Home Project. All the clinical strategic planning for the project was done by a multidisciplinary team that included representatives of nursing, medicine, occupational and recreational therapy, dietetics, physiotherapy, pharmacy, administration, chaplaincy, and volunteer services. Students participated freely in the project and reported that they felt more comfortable in their day-to-day dealings with these providers as a consequence of that participation (Rutgers College of Nursing, 1987). In this context, it should be noted that students' peer relationships are compromised when they participate on a team consisting of established providers rather than of students learning the discipline.

The complexity of practice increases as nurses participate in a workforce comprising workers with a variety of skill levels. In light of the growing number of chronically ill and frail elderly, it is clear that there are more and more lower-level activities in a therapeutic plan that cannot be accomplished through self-care and family care, but must nevertheless be done. The nursing shortage creates a further incentive to fill vacancies with nonprofessionals. Between 1980 and 1985, New Jersey dropped in rank from 15th to 32nd among the states with respect to the number of registered nurses per 1,000 hospital admissions (New Jersey State Nurses' Association, 1987). The absence of more detailed information makes it impossible to determine how much of this effect is due to substitution of nonprofessionals for registered nurses and how much is due to simple elimination of registered nurse positions. Even if it is assumed that this effect was due to some combination of these circumstances, it remains obvious that registered nurses are being expected to function with fewer traditional resources and to delegate activities to ancillary workers while still retaining responsibility. A quick interpretation might conclude that we are returning to outmoded models of supervision—layer on layer of people watching one another. Yet cost-consciousness is promoting new and better uses of the lesser skills of licensed practical nurses, nursing aides, volunteers, and even patients and their families.

Industrial psychology has created a large body of knowledge in human resource development. The modus operandi of this discipline is to work with people to encourage them to internalize the values that are held by the leader or philosophically established by the system. The system may be the client, the hospital, the home health agency, the primary nurse, or any combination of these. When subordinates understand and internalize these values, they require less supervision (Naisbitt & Aburdene, 1985). A natural first step toward helping others to internalize values is to clarify one's own values and one's own philosophy of care and ethical style. These insights should be developed in the educational program.

THE CLINICAL LABORATORY

In both the public and the private sector, reimbursement policy discourages the use of full-service residential programs such as hospitals and nursing homes. Community-based settings are a cost-efficient option that has not been adequately funded for either Medicare or Medicaid recipients; private-sector insurers have been more creative in reimbursing for community alternatives.

In exploring the implications for the nursing curriculum that stem from observations of the restructuring delivery system, we must distinguish between ambulatory and home health as settings for community care. Ambulatory care, including the burgeoning health market, has never been strategically or adequately developed by nursing. Home care, however, has historically been a bastion of nursing. Community practice could minimize some of the circumstances that have contributed significantly to the impoverished work environment in which nurses now find themselves: e.g., autonomy constraints, domination by physicians, and lack of direct access to clients. The Community Nursing Services and Ambulatory Care Act of 1987, presently before the 100th Congress, permits reimbursement to nurses under part B of Medicare without physician supervision or prescription (American Nurses' Association, 1987). The future looks bright for this legislation. If it is passed and implemented, it could establish community practice as an ideal employment setting for nurses.

The home health sector is currently in a stagnant, if not a deteriorating, condition. An ANA/AMA paper published at the beginning of the DRG era predicted a 300 percent increase in the volume of home care visits once the full effect of the Medicare prospective pricing system was felt (American Nurses' Association, 1984). This forecast relied on (1) the cost-efficiency of home care in comparison with hospitals or nursing homes; (2) the close connections between hospitals and community programs, which would enhance referrals; and (3) the need for continuing care created by early hospital discharge. Futurists failed, however, to anticipate the effect that public policy would have on the growth of home care. Medical and technical denials for home care services reimbursed through Medicare have increased dramatically since the DRG system was instituted, in October 1983. Denials increased from 18,121 in the last quarter of 1983 to 47,855 during the first quarter of 1986 (Senate Committee on Aging, 1986). Home care agencies have compromised themselves by becoming dependent on Medicare reimbursement and neglecting to diversify their services and sources of payment. In New Jersey, more than 75 percent of all home visits made during 1985 were made to elderly patients (New Jersey Home Health Assembly, 1987). Stringent definitions of "homebound" and "intermittent care" contribute significantly to the high rate of denial. Legislation sponsored by Senator Bill Bradley (D-New Jersey) promises to revise these criteria to make them more realistic. Changes in public policy could help revitalize home care.

The changing times have also created new hospital admission patterns. Same-day patients make up a significant cohort that is rarely referred to home care. Discharge planning is no longer properly integrated into the nursing role, and it does not progress at a pace that is compatible with the needs of the same-day patient. To a large extent, these patients are lost to aftercare. In our eagerness to adjust to increased acuity and reduce length of stay, we have sacrificed continuity, the aspect of nursing that ultimately has the greatest potential for cost savings.

We are left with the reality of a documented 37 percent increase in hospital discharges to home health care between 1983 and 1985, but only an 8 percent increase in Medicare visits for 1984. When we look more carefully at the nature of these visits, we see that even that modest increase offers little security for the future of nursing in home care. Data collected in New Jersey suggest that fewer and fewer of these visits involve registered nurses. Home care aides, technicians, and a vast variety of therapists dominate the home health care scene (Joel, 1985). It seems, therefore, that it is time for us to reconsider the questions of what manpower mix is appropriate to home care, how much supervision is necessary to safeguard the public, and who is to supervise whom.

Community health can only be reclaimed with the help of "the best and the brightest." To date, however, nurses have not found this practice setting particularly appealing. According to ANA statistics, in 1970 approximately 5 percent of employed nurses worked in community settings (excluding school nurses). By 1980 this figure had risen to 6.6 percent, but over the next five years it scarcely rose at all; in 1985, only 6.8 percent of nurses were employed in the community (Johnson, 1985). At this point, I should point out that most faculty, except for those who specialize in community or public health, have been socialized to hospital practice. Furthermore, community nursing has been depicted as a practice area that first requires experience in hospital practice. Faculty members convey these biases to students both subtly and directly.

We cannot deny the problems now apparent in community nursing, but we also cannot deny that the health care system, whether we like it or not, is moving in that direction. General hospitals report 50 million fewer inpatient days in 1986 than in 1981. The supply of acute care beds has been reduced by more than 40,000 since 1983 (Aiken & Mullinix, 1987). Regulations pending in New Jersey will adjust rates for the volume of inpatient admissions, thereby providing incentives for cost-efficient hospitals and eventually squeezing others out of business (New Jersey Health Care Administration Board, 1987).

In most educational programs, community nursing, in its broadest sense, receives at best token emphasis. Its situation is comparable to that of gerontologic nursing. Just as gerontologic nursing is more than caring for adults who happen to be a little older than average, community nursing is more than glorified home care. In both types of nursing, the predominant market and client of both today and tomorrow has been disenfranchised. To safeguard our future, the curriculum should provide a wide variety and a generous quantity of community experiences. The health market should be singled out for student experiences. Prejudices against using technical nurses in home care should be reassessed. Graduate preparation in community health should, out of necessity, require functional preparation for middle management.

Practicum diversification should not be limited to study of diverse clinical populations and settings. Whether by choice or by accident, we often fail to inform our students that many kinds of diversity are open to them in a nursing career. Nurses are for the most part salaried employees, and it seems likely that they will continue to be. Therefore, it becomes the responsibility of education to highlight the freedom and challenge that can be found or created in formal employment settings. The course of studies should introduce the opportunities available to intrapreneurs—that is, those risk-takers who approach invention within organized systems. Intrapreneurs refuse to relinquish the right to excitement simply because they are salaried employees (Naisbitt & Aburdene, 1985). They have a talent for negotiating highly complex systems, and they are skilled in finding and maximizing resources that the system affords and making the most of them (Pinchot, 1985). Nurses are excellent at systems negotiation; they have brought these talents to health care for generations. Such talents, which have only been documented informally, could be reinforced and strengthened by a systems orientation within the curriculum.

Furthermore, nurses need not commit their lives to direct patient care in order to contribute to the world of nursing. For example, their training makes them ideally suited to positions in utilization review and case coordination. They can make valuable contributions to government and organizational work. Many of these new opportunities can trace their origins to the advent of DRGs. Nurses are quick to criticize one another and even quicker to exclude those who dare to strike out in a nontraditional direction. Interest in an atypical nursing role is often misconstrued as failure to survive in nursing. This attitude must be combated. Nurses should be encouraged to pursue new roles, to claim them for nurses and nursing, and to use them as a platform for advocacy on behalf of their colleagues.

Examination of emergent practice roles, as I have described them in this chapter, suggests that the setting for clinical experiences may be less important than the role models provided and the role behaviors allowed. Faculty are not the role models for students, except in those rare instances in which faculty teach on their own panel of patients. Although faculty practice is the ultimate aim of many education-service collaborative efforts, this mission is often lost sight of over time. One of the most successful and most emotionally uplifting aspects of the Rutgers Teaching Nursing Home Project has been the rich learning experiences students gain from being directly assigned to registered nurses employed at the home. These nurses, who had a wide variety of entry-level preparations, were quick to allow students to test their clinical and management skills. They welcomed students' help in evaluating ancillary workers and in making decisions on appropriate delegation. At first, when students were offered a choice of clinical placements, they were reluctant to select a nursing home. Eventually, however, it became necessary to establish a waiting list for placement in the Teaching Nursing Home (Rutgers College of Nursing, 1987). Many students, looking back at their educational preparation, report that working in the Teaching Nursing Home was the clinical experience most relevant to their world of work.

The increasing acuity of hospital patients has also renewed interest in the use of service agency staff as preceptors to students. There is the constant assumption that faculty are on site and in control, but in practice it is almost impossible for a single instructor to supervise the activities of ten students who are taking care of extremely ill patients requiring highly complex care. In saying this, I do not mean to attack the 1:10 instructor:student ratio that is required by regulation in many states, merely to suggest that the use of staff as auxiliary teachers and preceptors should be maximized. Moreover, much of the art and science of clinical teaching lies in the case presentation and analysis that takes place in clinical pre- and post-conferences. I have observed that staff members rise to the occasion and profit psychologically, attitudinally, and technically from being selected to work with students (Patterson, 1987). Professionals have traditionally assumed responsibility for neophytes entering their field. In seeking to divorce ourselves from our roots, we have rejected many good aspects of apprenticeship education.

NEW BEHAVIORS FOR THE 1980s

The DRG system has started us along a path that allows less subjectivity and demands accountability from provider professionals. Personal accountability to the recipient of service has always been a hallmark of professionalism. Unfortunately, this quality became less common in the health care system as costs mushroomed and providers assumed ever greater dominance. Recent history reverses that pattern and places the consumer in a position of control. Professionals are being held accountable for their practices and in a sense for their colleagues' practices as well. Within nursing, this trend has been expressed through the growing tendency to decentralize clinical management decisions. The most familiar example is primary nursing.

To be fully responsible for oneself requires a practice autonomy and clarity of purpose that is frequently at odds with the role of the salaried professional. Proper socialization into accountability takes time and support. A commitment to peer review should be established early in the educational program, and peer review should be a regular component of clinical conferences. Students should continually evaluate one another as peers at similar levels of development. Every ministration and design element in care should be tracked to its ultimate outcome and evaluated against well-thought-out and comprehensive standards.

The standards against which to judge one's own practice are constantly changing. Often, the best or the only standard is one's own conscience. In the society of the future, adequacy in practice will depend on participation in an ongoing program of updating, a healthy respect for research, and access to a model for ethical decision making. It is respect for research that motivates staff nurses to incorporate new approaches to care into their clinical repertoire; it is the ethical orientation that directs them to weigh alternatives rather than act automatically. This openness to change and innovation first begins to be developed in an environment for learning that provides few answers and demands personal searches for truth. By now, we should have a good idea what kinds of research and ethical studies will help to foster such an environment. One way of enhancing these efforts might be to require students to carry out a self-guided review of the literature for a course instead of using a bibliography provided by faculty.

Nurses are personally responsible for the cost and efficacy of the care they deliver. Implicit in this statement are the strategies that will enable us to claim our market share of the delivery system: attaching a dollar value to our service, aiming for data-driven decisions, measuring outcomes, and documenting and establishing ownership of our contribution. Nurses have traditionally been uncomfortable with this degree of objectivity. Moreover, we have fallen into the habit of keeping inadequate records and are wary of broader applications of information processing. We must constantly remind ourselves, however, that nurses stand at the center of the health care system. They are the logical brokers of information, and in the future it is the providers with the most information and the best information who will move into positions of power and control. Consequently, it is time the curriculum paid attention to issues such as computer literacy. It is no secret that since the inception of DRGs, medical records has become the most powerful department in the hospital.

In the "information age" we live in, it is difficult for any curriculum to avoid becoming content-laden. Academic medicine and academic law have compensated for this difficulty by learning to think of process as content. In these disciplines, once the basic information is mastered, content is placed in a case orientation, and the focus of learning becomes problem-solving skills. The art of medical and legal education is to cultivate a professional approach to problem identification and resolution. Beyond accepting process as content, a highly conceptual curriculum can allow graduates to accommodate themselves more readily to rapid change in any scientific field.

Clearly, it becomes difficult to reconcile these educational principles with an employment setting that expects a confident practitioner. The gap between the conceptual and the concrete must be bridged by case-method simulations of clinical management and computer-assisted instruction. This gap is particularly wide and deep with respect to bioinstrumentation and medical devices. Nursing education programs have tended to minimize any obligation to develop technologic competence in their graduates. Many nurses never rise above an initial discomfort with technology and end up being controlled by it. This has led to the creation of new disciplines, such as bioengineers and technicians of various stripes. Problems with practice encroachment follow closely behind. These problems can only grow as technology spreads out from intensive care to find its way into the acute care unit, the nursing home, and the community. A relevant curriculum for the 1980s would include a heavy dose of physics and thorough review of equipment operating principles, frequent user errors, patient adverse reactions, common reasons for mechanical failure, and emergency operations.

A health care environment that is complex, unsettled, and to some degree hostile demands nurses who are assertive, strong in their practice, and steadfast in their convictions. Pioneers of this sort are necessary if nursing is to salvage its deteriorating and eroding markets for nursing and develop new ones. Personality testing to preselect occupational choices or provide counseling may be in the best interests of both the profession and the individual student. Much of nursing's current inability to capture more power and prestige is a direct result of its reluctance to accept expanded responsibility and its distaste for assertive action and unpleasantness.

We should remind ourselves that the nursing profession still has an exceptionally positive image among consumers. In a recent public opinion survey (ANA, 1985), consumers saw nurses as the group that could most logically expand their usual activities to help curtail health care costs. They also thought that nurses should be able to perform physical examinations and prescribe medications. It seems that nurses have far more reservations about their skills and abilities than their clients do. If in the late 1980s, when professionals in all categories have lost much of the respect they were once accorded by society, we still have maintained a good image; we would be remiss not to take steps to capitalize on that situation immediately. Anyone who scans the press knows that we may soon lose this consumer edge. Articles in magazines and newspapers not uncommonly attribute hospital fatalities and inadequate health care to the absence of seasoned and experienced nurses ("New York Hospital on the Spot," 1987). Reports like these, if not countered, will begin to chip away at the good reputation of the profession. It remains to be seen whether nursing would fare better if candidates to the field were selected for their risk-taking capacity and interpersonal effectiveness.

Acceptance of the responsibilities I have described demands the qualities of a professional. This being the case, socialization into role may be the single most important goal of education. The more established professions have built a concentrated study of the discipline on the foundation of a liberal education. A similar preprofessional course of studies that emphasizes the natural and behavior sciences and the humanities may be the best preparation for the intense study of nursing. Immersion in professional studies to the exclusion of elective and supportive courses may facilitate the development of professional identity. The professions of law and medicine have been successful in developing identity, self-esteem, and collegiality among their members. The nature and length of the preprofessional sequence holds both educational and political implications. The preprofessional requirement could be two years (an associate degree) or the baccalaureate, with a master's degree as the educational credential for entry into professional practice. (The precise nature of the requirement should, of course, be determined by discussion and debate.) Ultimately, we may find that the restructuring of health care requires fewer but more sophisticated nurses.

The process of socialization into role is closely associated with the transition to practice that the student inevitably faces. The pain and disillusionment that frequently accompany this transition are well known. Nursing has traditionally made very little allowance for the insecurity of the new graduate. Creative approaches to easing the transition from student to professional should be formally endorsed by nursing education. Work-study programs (assuming that the work is nursing) create a comfort with practice. Academically endorsed placement of students with affiliate agencies for summer work and part-time employment during the school year are other options. Making postgraduate residencies or externships part of the educational program should also be considered. Such new approaches raise many questions. Should they be mandatory or optional? Who should control the program, education or service? Should participants be compensated?

CONCLUSIONS

The state of health care in the 1980s invites nurses to assume a more vigorous and visible leadership role. Health care has become more complex, and service gaps exist that compromise cost-efficiency. Nurses are uniquely suited to fix what is wrong by applying their talents to integrating, coordinating, and developing human resources and to acting as client advocates. Acquisition of middle management skills, a research attitude, the ability to create and process information, and comfort with advanced technology will allow nursing to claim its market share of the delivery system. There are numerous opportunities that could attract "the brightest and the best" into nursing.

The entry-level curriculum should establish the ethos of personal accountability for one's own practice, for the practice of ancillary personnel, and, in the broadest sense, for the practice of one's colleagues. Conscious acceptance of this responsibility will bring nurses one step closer to controlling the practice environment instead of being controlled by it.

The rapid expansion of technology and the limited shelf-life of knowledge are a challenge to all the applied sciences. The implications for nursing curricula are significant. A course of studies should consist of content that is selective, conceptual, and process-oriented. Educators must resist the temptation to "teach it all." Clinical material should rarely be used for its own sake; rather, it should be used as a vehicle for developing the cognitive processes that characterize the professional.

The challenges I have detailed demand the development of a truly *professional* practice, while recognizing that an assisting role also exists. It is critical to move on from nursing's educational agenda of the past two decades. The times demand that organized nursing rise above internal politics to upgrade its practice and to standardize its educational requirements for entry into the field.

REFERENCES

Aiken, L. H., & Mullinix, C. F. (1987). The nursing shortage. *The New England Journal of Medicine, 317* (10), 641–645.

American Nurses' Association. (1984, September). *ANA's concerns regarding the impact of the prospective financing mechanisms on nursing service*. Kansas City, MO: Author.

American Nurses' Association. (1987). *Introduction of community nursing organizations legislation*. Washington, DC: Author.

American Nurses' Association. (1985). *National public opinion survey on nursing*. Kansas City, MO: Author.

DeMaio, D. (1979). Born again nurse. *Nursing Outlook, 27* (4), 272–273.

Joel, L. (1985). *Nursing's role in the changing health scene*. Seattle: University of Washington School of Nursing.

Joel. L. (1987). Reshaping nursing practice. *American Journal of Nursing, 87* (6), 793–795.

Johnson, C. (1985, October). Personal communication.

Lang, N. (1987, September). Keynote address delivered at the Annenberg Conference on Nursing in the 21st Century, Palm Springs, CA.

Middle Atlantic Regional Nursing Association (MARNA). (1987). *Survey of curriculum adaptations in response to the DRG system*. Unpublished report.

Naisbitt, J., & Aburdene, P. (1985). *Reinventing the corporation*. New York: Warner Books.

New Jersey Department of Health. (1984). *Hospital management reports*. Trenton, NJ: Author.

New Jersey Health Care Administration Board. (1987). Minutes of public meeting, November 13, 1987.

New Jersey Home Health Assembly. (1987). *1985 Home Health Data*. Princeton, NJ: Author.

New Jersey State Nurses' Association. (1987). *Quality health care in New Jersey . . . the nurses' perspective*. Trenton, NJ: Author.

New York Hospital on the Spot. (1987, June). *New York Magazine*, pp. 40– 47.

Patterson, J. (1987). Maximizing RN potential in a long-term care setting. *Geriatric Nursing, 8* (3), 142–144.

Pinchot, G. (1985). *Intrapreneuring*. New York: Harper & Row.

Rutgers College of Nursing, Teaching Nursing Home Project. (1987). Final report. Unpublished report.

Rutigliano, A. J. (1985). Surgery on health care costs. *Management Review, 85* (10), 25–32.

Senate Committee on Aging. (1986). *The crisis in home health care: Greater need, less care*. Washington, DC: US Senate.

3

New Directions for a New Age

Em Olivia Bevis

I often cynically think that curriculum development is something one does to keep from getting bored with teaching the same way every time and something administration uses to keep the faculty busy. I feel this way because most curriculum development results in minimal changes of substance. Usually we negotiate a new philosophy or polish up an old one; we reconceptualize, theorize, and agonize some concepts and theories we want to emphasize; we integrate, irritate or deteriorate our program objectives; we switch, swap, and slide content around; we rename, malign, and design a new program of studies; we refine and realign our course outlines; and we develop evaluation tools to assess whether or not students have met the designated behaviors. Then we open the champagne and celebrate that it is over—over, that is, until a new curriculum coordinator or dean is hired and we start again. Sometimes I feel much as the great Roman philosopher/orator Seneca wrote in his *Epistles* almost 2,000 years ago: "I was shipwrecked before I got aboard."

The very repetitiveness of our curriculum development efforts should be telling us that we are not changing the substance, only the arrangement of content. In order to change the substance, to alter the type of graduate, to graduate a professional, to create a true discipline of nursing, we must have a revolution that attacks the basic tenets of nursing curriculum development; that deinstitutionalizes the Tyler curriculum model and its mandated products; that makes nursing philosophy, research, and education congruent; that distinguishes between learning that is training and learning that is education; that alters our perception of teaching and the role of the teacher; that abandons the industrial metaphor; that restructures the relative roles of classroom and clinical practice; that de-emphasizes curriculum development and concentrates on faculty development; that develops a national strategy for change; and, above all, that provides new guideposts for a new age.

I have written this paper as a manifesto in the sense defined by Webster: as a public declaration of intentions, motives or views, a public statement of policy or opinion. Its aim, while certainly difficult to realize, can be simply put: to initiate the type of curriculum revolution in nursing education described above. It will contain a brief history of curriculum development in nursing so that we gain some perspective about where we are, with a comprehensive examination of the strengths and limitations of our present curriculum development model. And, in the real sense of a manifesto, it will specify what must become our public policy in order to bring about a new age, the age of nursing as a true discipline and as a profession—policies that must be established if our revolution is to succeed.

BRIEF HISTORY

To date there have been four turns in nursing curriculum development and one, I believe, that must come. (See Figure 1.) The first, which Isobel Stewart (1947) called "the first hopeful step toward reform," came in the 17th century from the French Sisters of Charity. A part of that same turn was initiated by the Deaconesses at Kaiserwerth in the 19th century.

The second turn in curriculum development occurred in 1860 and was, of course, due to the efforts of the founder of modern nursing, Florence Nightingale. Enough has been written about the school at St. Thomas that I need not belabor it here. However, I cannot resist telling you that in examining that curriculum (Nightingale, 1867) I found that, in addition to 13 mandatory areas of skill, students were required to be sober, honest, truthful, trustworthy, punctual, quiet and orderly, cleanly [sic] and neat, patient, cheerful, and kindly. (I presume at the end of this you were sainted instead of graduated.)

The third turn in curriculum came with the publication of the *Standard Curriculum for Schools of Nursing* prepared by the Education Committee of the League of Nursing Education in 1917. It was described as an "optimum" curriculum so that schools could voluntarily improve

Figure 1
Five Turns in Nursing Curriculum

	First Turn
17th Century	French Sisters of Charity
19th Century	German Deconesses at Kaiserswerth
	Second Turn
1860	Florence Nightingale, the School at St Thomas
	Third Turn
1917	The Standard Curriculum for Schools of Nursing
1927	A Curriculum for Schools of Nursing
1937	Curriculum Guide for Schools of Nursing
	The Education Committee of the National League of Nursing Education
	Fourth Turn
1950	Ralph Tyler: Basic Principles of Curriculum and Instruction
	Fifth Turn
1987	The Curriculum Revolution: Models Emphasizing Teaching in a Practice Discipline

their programs. It came about at a time when state requirements were minimal and not at all uniform. This book provided objectives, content, and methods for each course and listed materials, equipment, and bibliographies. It even provided a schedule for operating a school on an eight-hour plan. The objectives were not the prescriptive behavioral objectives we have grown accustomed to today, but more in the line of general and specific goals. It was revised in 1927 and again in 1937 under the title of *Curriculum Guide for Schools of Nursing*. World War II came along and so changed nursing that this book was allowed to go out of print.

It was more than a decade before another book was published that instigated the fourth turn in nursing curriculum, Ralph Tyler's course syllabus on curriculum development.

However, a great deal of progress not associated with curriculum development models has been made in the time span from 1940 to the present. Not a little of this progress has been the movement of nursing education from hospital-based training programs to academic settings. As early as 1898, university courses for graduate nurses were developed at Columbia University Teachers College. Then the first real, totally collegiate school was created in 1909 when the University of Minnesota "put the whole school of nursing connected with its university hospital on a dignified standing as a professional school of the university" (Dock & Stewart, 1925). Beginning in the 1940s, literally hundreds of college and university schools of nursing opened. A second educational factor that greatly influenced nursing practice was the experiment by Mildred Montag (1951) of placing nursing curriculum in two-year colleges. In doing this, she followed the advice of several study groups (Goldmark, 1923) and nursing educational experts (Brown, 1948; Wolf, 1947). As you know, she designed a two-year course of study for "technical nurses." Based upon Montag's model, two-year colleges all over the nation developed associate of arts degree nursing programs, gradually filling the slot in the health care scene held by hospital diploma programs. One benefit of this movement was that it brought most nursing education into institutions of higher learning.

The demise of the 1937 *Curriculum Guide* left a vacuum that was filled by the 1950 publication of the Tyler curriculum development model. This, as mentioned, was the fourth and current turn in curriculum development. Essentially, this school of thought maintains that all curriculum development, regardless of the nature of the process used, must result in certain prescribed curriculum outcomes. (See Figure 2.) These outcomes or products of curriculum development are: a philosophy; a conceptual framework (introduced as such by Taba, 1962); behaviorally defined, measurable objectives on every level (program, curriculum, course, unit or module, and learning activity); the development or selection of learning activities sorted into a program of studies;

Figure 2
Prescribed Curriculum Development Products of the Tyler-Type Models

1. A Philosophy
2. Concepts/Threads/Strands/Theoretical Constructs (conceptual framework)
3. Program objectives (behaviorally defined and measurable)
4. Level objectives (behaviorally defined and measurable)
5. Program of studies
6. Course objectives (behaviorally defined and measurable)
7. Unit or Module objectives (behaviorally defined and measurable)
8. Learning activity objectives (behaviorally defined and measurable)
9. Behaviorally defined and measurable criteria for student evaluation

and the evaluation of learning based on the behavioral objectives. The authorities may vary in their definition of curriculum, the order and sequence of the prescribed developmental steps, and the components or the content of the development steps; but they all agree on the above products.

In 1955, Ole Sand published the report of three years of action research in curriculum revision conducted at the University of Washington School of Nursing. This book substantiated the practicality of using the Tyler rationale to develop nursing curriculum. Since Ralph Tyler was consultant to the project, it is not surprising that the methodology of curriculum development used and, therefore, recommended to American nursing educators was the Tyler model. The book became a replacement for the now out-of-print *Curriculum Guide* and the Tyler rationale gradually became institutionalized by state boards of nursing and the National League for Nursing. These powerful agencies, through the use of regulations, criteria, and the way site visitors were oriented, made it mandatory to use the Tyler curriculum development products for every one of the wide variety of types of non-doctoral programs in nursing: diploma, associate of arts, baccalaureate, and master's. The obvious consequence of this forced "sameness" in curriculum development models was some degree of similarity in the graduates. It was, and remains, very difficult to differentiate among graduates of the three most popular types of programs. While I am not willing to suggest that the mandated sameness in the curriculum development model is the single cause for this (nothing is that simple), certainly the utilization of the same curriculum development model, and that one a technical or training model, is a major factor.

There were two additional forces that affirmed the Tyler-type curriculum development products as nursing curriculum dogma. The first and most obvious was my book on curriculum development, which played no small part in confirming the Tyler-type behaviorist technical model as *the* model for nursing. It served its purpose, but it is time to move forward. The second force that helped reduce a curriculum development model to nursing curriculum dogma was Mager's (1962) book, *Preparing Instructional Objectives*. Soon after its publication, workshops were held all across the United States to insure that every nurse educator had an opportunity to attend sessions to learn to write and use "measurable, behavioral objectives" correctly. The reverence for behavioral objectives reached such a peak (and remains there) that even their development has become formula-driven and rigid.

STRENGTHS OF THE TYLER MODEL

I cannot join the critics that would blame the Tyler rationale for all of nursing's curriculum troubles, for it has had a positive impact on the quality of nursing education. During the post-World War II period, there was a veritable explosion of health care that accompanied the general expansion of technology and education. Nursing education entered a phase of growth in both quantity and quality.

The strict insistence on measurable behavioral objectives backed by force of law, custom, and accreditation focused the training and instructional aspects of nursing in such a way as to help lift it to a highly organized, evaluation-oriented, and regulated group that provides services of reliable quality. Along with improved laws governing schools, licensure, and excellent accreditation procedures, schools of nursing have attained a quality seen in few other disciplines. They have an unusual ability to monitor and police themselves and a sense of responsibility and commitment to the public trust that is not found in any of the other like groups, medical, legal or clerical. Tyler's curriculum development products provided the tools to be used in the search for quality, and then, sadly, they became ends in themselves.

THE CASE FOR A REVOLUTION

It is obvious to all of us here, since the title of this conference is a "Curriculum Development Revolution," that one of the problems facing us is that nursing education is currently bogging down. It is encountering increasing problems in moving nursing further along the professional continuum. The "well educated," critical-thinking nursing professional emerges infrequently from colleges and universities.

There are many reasons for this. Bloom (1987), in his recent book, *The Closing of the American Mind,* would blame it on relativism. I think it is much more than that. Some other etiologies are: the falling quality of high school graduates; the attraction of good students to other professions and occupations; the inadequate time for providing a liberal arts education simultaneously with a professional one; and the paucity of well-educated teachers. Each of these requires our attention. Some are extrinsic factors over which we have relatively little control. Most we can affect in small ways. However, the one I think most critical, and over which we do have control, is the use of the Tyler model for curriculum development. I feel compelled, therefore, to criticize that model as a basis for my proposals for change. I believe that until we do something to abolish the use of the Tyler model as the *exclusively* sanctioned model for curriculum development in nursing, nothing else will be successful in moving us into our new age of professionalism. (See Figure 3.)

Criticism of the Tyler Model

My first criticism is this: the Tyler model is based in behaviorist-learning theory, and behaviorism lends itself to training, not to education.

Since Tyler-type models are the only sanctioned models in nursing, they are used for all curriculum development without ascertaining whether or not other models exist that might be better for some levels of nursing education. What is helpful to some of the technical or training aspects of nursing is a liability when used for developing the professional level of curriculum. In other words, generic education, which is the initial nursing education leading to licensure, has some content that lends itself to behaviorism and, therefore, to training. However, behaviorism does not permit education. And as one moves up the educational ladder toward and through baccalaureate, master's, and doctoral education, behaviorism becomes devastatingly limiting.

Regardless of what one's philosophy and conceptual framework state about beliefs in learning and learning theory, as long as behavioral objectives are used as the sole guides for selecting and devising learning activities and as long as they are the sole source of evaluation of student learning, the *de facto* learning theory of every school is behaviorism and, therefore, the focus is on training in the technical aspects of nursing.

Behavioral objectives as the sole arbiters of learning are too narrow and lack the creative energy necessary to guide the awakening discov-

Figure 3
Criticism: The Case for Revolution

1. The current model is based in behaviorist learning theory and behaviorism lends itself to training, not to education.
2. Behavioral objectives are too narrow and lack the creative energy necessary to guide the awakening discovery that must mark true education.
3. Behavioral objectives, by their nature, obviate education.
4. A curriculum development model cannot be the dictator of our educational progress and our response to the societal mandate.

ery that must mark true education. Behavioral objectives represent minimal achievement levels, and are effective primarily for skill training and instruction. But they are not useful for seeing patterns and finding meanings, for enculturation into the profession or for learning the creative strategies necessary to identify, classify, and solve the problems of the discipline. They stifle creativity and provide restrictive guides for evaluations. When one remembers that under the objectives model, evaluation and grading have become the power that drives teaching rather than learning (which should be the energy source), one can see how restrictive behavioral objectives are. If used exclusively—and, again, the Tyler-type technical curriculum development models currently are the only sanctioned models—they become inhibitors to achieving the very essence of professional education.

Essentially, behavioral objectives identify the concrete, measurable behaviors that the faculty perceives as important, ignoring the students' values, interests, and natural bent. Because of the nature of the legitimate objectives, teachers cannot facilitate the achievement of goals that are not empirically verifiable. Behavioral objectives are congruent with a philosophy of empiricism but out of step with humanistic-existential goals and nursing as a human science.

Behavioral objectives by their very nature negate education. Kleibard (1970) puts it very strongly:

> From a moral point of view, the emphasis on behavioral goals, despite all of the protestations to the contrary, still borders on brainwashing or at least indoctrination rather than education. We begin with some notion of how we want a person to behave and then we try to manipulate him and his environment so as to get him to behave as we want him to.

He is correct. Further, creativity, individualization, independent thinking, criticism, reflection, identifying and evaluating assumptions, inquiry into the nature of things, projecting, futuring, predicting, searching for patterns, or motifs that organize the mind, viewing wholes, internalizing paradigm experiences, and finding personal meanings are not consequences of behaviorist training.

Along these same lines, Watson (1979) offers the following criticism:

> Nursing is becoming established as an academic discipline that requires a liberal arts education. It is therefore incumbent on the profession and the academic community to adhere to the purpose of a university education—to gain knowledge and understanding. More energy is now expended in the acquisition of scientific knowl-

> edge than of understanding. Nursing tries to understand people and how they cope with health and illness.
>
> [nursing] tries to understand how health and illness and human behavior are interrelated. Nursing education rarely concentrates on that level of understanding. In some ways nursing schools are still technical, professional schools. Many teachers and schools state attempts to develop self-actualization. However, they end up hidden, primarily teaching specialized terminology, procedures, scientific principles, the basic content of behavior, pathophysiology, and the disease processes. (pp. 2–3)

A curriculum development model cannot be the dictator of our educational progress and the guide to our response to society's mandate. In nursing, Tyler has become less a guide for curriculum development and more a legal code. His curriculum development products have been translated into essential components. Without evidence of these there can be no approval by state boards of nursing nor accreditation by the National League for Nursing. Therefore, if a school does not follow the Tyler-type curriculum development models and cannot show the products of these models, its graduates are not allowed to take licensure examinations and its program will not be accredited. That is institutionalization at its most powerful. Our social mandate is such that it demands care that can only be given by educated professionals.

THE MANIFESTO: GUIDELINES FOR THE NEW AGE

Based on these criticisms, it becomes apparent that we must depart from the Tyler model. We must do more than that, but we must first begin with changing the sanctity of Tyler. In order to usher in a new age for nursing, we must work together to establish a new "public policy" for nursing. The change must occur as a totality. It must be organismic. It would be an insidious sabotage of the curriculum revolution to allow even one of our pet ideas to exist unexamined and uncriticized. To that end, I offer the following suggestions.

The first will come as no surprise to you considering the groundwork I have laid.

Deinstitutionalize the Tyler Curriculum Development Model

Nursing's use of the Tyler rationale for approval and accreditation was never intended by Tyler. It was designed for use as a "guide," not as a code—laws so immutable as to make the Ten Commandments easier to break without bringing down organized condemnation and punitive consequences. The Tyler-type curriculum development products have come to constitute nursing educational dogma, creating a frighteningly single-track educational prescription that ignores all aspects of education not covered by behaviors and *finite*, preconceived, measurable outcomes. This has, as a consequence, a curriculum as inadequate as it is limited in its conception and its implementation. It leaves as irrelevant the large mass of learned aptitudes that are not measurable. It discounts insights, analysis, and patterns. It discards any and all joy taken by the student in the private world of discovery, in the walk alone through the peaks and valleys of the student's own mind. It ignores what Watson (1985) calls "soul," a term she defines as the "spirit, inner self, or essence of the person, which is tied to a greater sense of self-awareness, a higher degree of consciousness, an inner strength, and a power that can expand human capacities and allow a person to transcend his or her usual self" (p. 46). It ignores insights and learnings that incubate in the time capsule of the mind to emerge years later like the Goddess of wisdom, Pallas, Athene, fully armed from the brow of Zeus, to tackle some obscure enigma.

To remain with the Tyler behaviorist, technical model of curriculum development is to ignore the higher levels of thought processes that are educative and to discard or place in peril the professionalism for which all nurses strive.

Behaviorism can produce efficient nurses on a technical level; the long, successful use of behavioral objectives has proved this beyond any doubt. It can be used in professional levels of education for those aspects of nursing that are training. What it cannot do is support the changes necessary to keep pace with society's changing demands and the natural evolution of nursing into a discipline and a profession. It has not been able to do this for a long time now, and most educators know it. (See Figure 4.)

Figure 4
The Three Types of Curriculum

1. The legitimate curriculum—training; technical
2. The illegitimate curriculum—educative; mostly syntactical
3. The hidden curriculum—socialization; mostly contextual

Therefore, every school has three curricula:

1. The legitimate curriculum: the one agreed on by the faculty in their long sessions and debates, written into plans and sanctioned by the approval and accreditation bodies.
2. The illegitimate curriculum: the one kept in the closet, that we all know is there, that we teach quite openly but cannot grade because this curriculum of insights, patterns, creativity, strategies, and understanding does not fit behavioral objectives.
3. The hidden curriculum: the one we are unaware of and which appears in the way we teach the priorities we set, the type of methods we use, and the way we interact with students. This is the curriculum of subtle socialization, of teaching initiates how to think and feel like nurses.

So we have three curricula, the legitimate, the illegitimate, and the hidden. Currently in nursing the legitimate curriculum is behaviorist. Being training-oriented and technical, it cannot support professionalism and is useful only for the technical aspects of nursing. *The professional aspects of curriculum demand that it be abandoned.* To this end, we must prevail upon the National League for Nursing and the National Council of State Boards of Nursing to support deinstitutionalization. In evaluating nursing curriculum, emphasis must not be limited to the existence of a philosophy, identified theories, behavioral objectives on every level, and behavioral objective-driven student evaluation. Instead, we must find ways to assess the merit of programs based on the two most critical curriculum factors: (1) the quality of, or the educational nature of, the learning activities and (2) the effectiveness of teacher-student interactions for fostering education.

Rather than institutionalize another model to replace the Tyler type, we must become aware of the several models now evolving. I have developed a "Professional or Educative Model." Nancy Diekelmann has developed a "Dialogue and Meaning Model." Certainly there are others I do not know about. Since we do not want to replace one dogma with another, we must allow schools to choose or develop models that satisfy their particular needs. We must not be afraid of innovation and difference. We need only fear Emerson's "hobgoblin of little minds": a foolish consistency.

Make Congruent Nursing Philosophy, Research, and Education

Already the philosophical basis of nursing is shifting. Munhall (1982), in her classic article, "Nursing Research, in Apposition or Opposition," raised questions regarding the assumptions on which nursing research was based and pointed out how nursing philosophy had evolved along a different pathway. Her identification of the assumptions underlying empiricist research methodology could well be applied to nursing curriculum. Nursing education is also in opposition to nursing's philosophical base and, like research, has continued to be driven by empiricist philosophy. I am recommending that, as in nursing research, qualitative as well as quantitative methods be used and that empiricism in the guise of behaviorism not be the only driver of nursing curriculum. Empiricist philosophy manifests itself most clearly in Thorndike's famous assertion that everything that exists, exists in some quantity and, therefore, can be measured. Under this rubric it is quite natural that learning be defined as a change in behavior and that if there is no change in behavior, learning has not occurred.

Distinguish Between Learning That is Training and Learning That is Education

It becomes clear, then, that in our curriculum revolution the third aspect we must change is our perception of what learning is, so that training is distinguished from education in ways that give education decisive power in the curriculum.

The development of learning theory seems to have been undertaken with the assumption that a pan theory could be devised that would serve for all learning. Learning theorists advocate one theory over another, and hostilities among antagonists both amuse and bemuse those who struggle to teach. Teachers discover very quickly that all learning theories work depending upon what one is teaching.

The problem arises when teachers, in dealing with reality, find that for some learning situations and problems one theory works better than another. This suggests that there are distinct types of learning and these types are substantively different. If one took a different assumption—for instance, that there are different types of learning—then it would follow that various theories of learning may be more appropriate or relevant to one type than to another. Therefore, to begin our "New Age," I have examined nursing content and used that analysis to type learning and to distinguish among types those that are training (technical) and those that are educational (professional).

The typology suggested here assumes that type of content is directly related to learning types, and that people learn different types of content differently. A student does not memorize a list of medical vocabulary and abbreviations in the same way he or she learns to innovate nursing care strategies for a patient with difficult problems. Carried to another level, it seems appropriate to define learning differently according to the various types. (Note that I am not defining learning here.)

Typing learning so that training can be differentiated from education helps teachers know the kind of learning activities to develop and the kind of questions to raise with students in their interactions. Botkin, Elmandjra, and Malitza (1979), Raths (1971), Stenhouse (1980), Schwab (1979), Eisner (1982), and many others suggest that one goes about training differently from educating. It follows, therefore, that these differences can be accounted for by assuming that there are entirely different types of learning involved.

If several types of learning do exist, then these could be used, among other things, as a means of sorting content, of differentiating between technical and professional education, and of differentiating among levels of professional education.

Since distinctions between training and education are necessary to all "New Age" curriculum models, brief descriptions of each of the six types of learning and their uses follow.* (See Figure 5.)

1. *Item learning* deals with learning separate pieces of information, individual factors and simple relationships (e.g., lists and procedures), and the use of tools and equipment (e.g., catheters and monitors). It deals with acquiring the ability to complete a task mechanically and ritualistically; for example, how to take a temperature and appropriate sites for taking it.

2. *Directive learning* is specifically concerned with rules, injunctions, and exceptions to rules. It deals with the "do's" and "don'ts" regarding tasks. This type of learning includes the assembling of items into a *safe* system of directions. By necessity, directive learning follows item learning or can be learned concurrently; for example, when and when not to take an oral temperature.

3. *Rational learning* uses theory to buttress practice. It provides the rationale for why one nursing intervention is better than another. It enables the learner to study rationales and the use of theories in practice. It is characterized by arranging items and directions in some logical order, and finding theories to inform practice (or, if you prefer, on which to base practice). It addresses the logical use of *formal* properties

*This material was developed in collaboration with Tamar Bermann, Chief Researcher, Work Research Institutes, Oslo, Norway

Figure 5
Types of Learning

1. *ITEM LEARNING*: separate pieces of information, individual factors and simple relationships such as lists, procedures, using tools and equipment. It is mechanical and ritualistic.
2. *DIRECTIVE LEARNING*: rules, injunctions, and exceptions; the "do's" and "don'ts" regarding tasks. It is assembling items into a *safe* system of directions.
3. *RATIONAL LEARNING*: uses theory to buttress or inform practice. Addresses why one nursing intervention is better than another. It is characterized by logical arrangements of the items and directions, addresses the logical use of *formal* properties and theories, and enables learners to relate information, feelings, ideas, and plans to skills. It exerts influence on judgment and decision making, and enables the learner to apply research to practice.
4. *SYNTACTICAL LEARNING*: seeing meaningful wholes, relationships and patterns; departure from rule-driven care; providing individualized, unique client care with care models that are grounded in practice-supporting personal guides and paradigms; addresses the lived moment and the relationships that ideas, concepts, and theories have with each other; consequential reasoning and substantive views of relationships; having insights and finding meanings. This type enables people to make intuitive leaps and to trust them, and helps weld together theory and practice to support praxis.
5. *CONTEXTUAL LEARNING*: culturality; the mores, folkways, rites, rituals and accepted ways of being a nurse; the language and other symbols of nursing; political expertise in the profession and its use; power and its use; work role relationships; values, esthetics, ethics, and philosophy. This type influences nurses' transactions with clients and with colleagues so that these transactions are caring, compassionate, and positive.
6. *INQUIRY LEARNING*: creativity; investigation, theorizing, strategizing, identifying, clarifying and categorizing problems and approaches to solving them. It is idea generating: leaping into new dimensions; posing questions, formulating positions, fantasizing new ways, alterations that improve things and systems; projecting, futuring, predicting from knowns to unknowns using both data and intuition; visualizing possibilities, dreaming dreams, having visions, and devising ways to make real these possible realities. It is seeing assumptions that are behind positions and questioning their validity; seeing beyond words to their implications and applications and enjoying the quest as much as the success.

of activities and theories, and enables the learner to relate information, feelings, ideas, and plans to skills. It exerts influence on judgment and decision making, and enables the learner to apply research to practice; for example, focus would be directed to the physiological rationale of why a nurse would not take an oral temperature soon after the client has had a drink of cold water.

These first three types of learning strategies aid in the training of nurses and are the focus of technical nursing programs only.

4. *Syntactical learning* is characterized by the logical structure or arrangement of data into meaningful wholes, and will influence how a nurse uses all other types of learning. The qualities of circumstances are used in ways that enable departure from rule-driven interventions or responses and to a provision of care that is individualized to unique client situations. The use of formal and informal properties and the ability to relate experiences to care are of concern here.

Syntactical learning is finding patterns, examples, and models that are grounded in practice and that support formation of personal general guides and paradigms. It also provides the nurse with an understanding of when and under what circumstances to depart from these guides and paradigms. It addresses the lived moment; the relationships that ideas, concepts, and theories have with each other in practical usage. Such consequential reasoning and substantive views of relationships are characterized by viewing wholes, having insights, and finding meanings. It provides the reality and structure for evaluation. Syntactical learning enables nurses to make intuitive leaps and to trust them. It helps weld together theory and practice in such a way that actual praxis exists. High levels of learning in this category make the experts described by Benner (1984).

The foundations of syntactical learning are laid in generic baccalaureate programs, but real syntactical learning is seldom attained without experience or a master's clinical specialization. An example of syntactical learning would be the quick clinical insight necessary to know not to waste three to five minutes taking a temperature on a child but to move quickly to head off a convulsion that will be the inevitable consequence of a child's high fever.

5. *Contextual learning* is the interrelated conditions in which the discipline and its practice exist or occur. It is the essence of nursing. It is learning the things that characterize nursing and make it unique. Contextual learning focuses on the socio-cultural context of the discipline: the mores, folkways, rites, rituals, and accepted ways of being a nurse. It helps the learner think and feel like a nurse. It encompasses the language and other symbols of nursing. It is the development of political expertise in the profession and it is used in health agencies, in government, and in education to shape policy and legislation. It is, in other words, the acquisition of power and its use. Contextual learning deals with the relationships in the work roles of coordination, collaboration, and colleagueship. It is learning the values, esthetics, ethics, and general philosophy of nursing. It is learning to perceive nursing as a human science in ways that influence nurses' transactions with clients and

with colleagues so that these transactions are caring, compassionate, and positive.

6. *Inquiry learning* is the creative aspect of nursing. It is the art of investigation, the search for truth, the generation of theory. Strategizing is the main theme in this category. It contains materials that help nurses learn how to identify, clarify, and categorize problems and ways or approaches to solving the problems of nursing as it attempts to be responsive to the society it serves. Further, it is idea generating: leaping creatively into new dimensions, posing questions, formulating positions, fantasizing new ways to improve things and systems; projecting, futuring, predicting from knowns to unknowns using both data and intuition; visualizing possibilities, dreaming dreams, having visions, and devising ways to make real these possible realities. In this category the nurse learns to see assumptions that are behind positions and to question their validity, to see beyond words to their implications and applications, and to enjoy the quest as much as the success.

Earlier I mentioned the use of this typology in researching differences in types of programs. To do that, a nurse would need to examine curricula to determine the degree of training or education addressed in each type of program. The three tables that follow are the result of an experiential guess at what we would find.

Table 1 illustrates which types of learning are training and which are education. If true, this provides some direction for differentiating among technical and professional education.

What must be noted here is that all generic programs, including the generic master's and doctorate, contain some training. Some nursing content must be memorized, and rules for the use of certain skills and their underlying rationales must be learned. However, the amounts of training in technical programs would differ from professional ones.

Table 2 presents a rough estimate of the types of learning included in the various curriculum development models in existence today. The generic master's and doctorate programs are not addressed specifically but, because of their generic nature, would probably fall somewhere

Table 1
Technical and Professional Content by Types of Learning

	Item	Direct	Rational	Syntactical	Contextual	Inquiry
Technical	X	X	X			
Professional				X	X	X

Table 2
Estimated Percentage of Type of Learning Currently in Nursing Curricula by Type of Program

	Item	Direct	Rational	Syntactical	Contextual	Inquiry
Practical	60	27	10	0	3	0
Diploma	35	30	17	3	15	0
Associate	35	30	17	3	10	5
Baccalaureate	25	25	20	5	15	10
Masters	5	5	20	25	30	35
Doctorate	0	0	5	10	15	70

between baccalaureate and master's degree programs. The increased amount of humanities and other liberal arts courses allowed by the generic doctorate would probably enable a greater use of contextual and inquiry learning.

Percentages are not the only elements affected by alterations in programs. For instance, in contextual learning, the very nature of the content included in the program may differ. Diploma education and baccalaureate education may both have contextual (socialization) content, but the nature of the content chosen for the overt curriculum or existing in the hidden curriculum may vary considerably. The American Association of Colleges of Nursing's (AACN) (1986) final report on the "Essentials of College and University Education for Professional Nursing" posits that "Values are reflected in attitudes, personal qualities, and consistent patterns of behaviors." And they go on to recommend seven values that are deemed essential for the professional nurse: altruism, equality, esthetics, freedom, human dignity, justice, and truth. All of these fall into the category called here "contextual" and in the AACN report "socialization." Such values are probably inherent in all nursing programs regardless of level. However, the content chosen and the socialization aspects in the hidden curriculum would emphasize different aspects of these values and place more or less stress upon them. It would not be true that technical programs do not teach these values in either the overt or the hidden curricula.

Table 3 illustrates an estimate of the percentage of types of learning in nursing programs if educative curriculum development models were used.

The baccalaureate and master's programs are predicted to alter in

Table 3
Estimated Percentage of Type of Learning in Nursing Curricula by Type of Program if Educative (Professional) (Non-Behaviorist) Curriculum Development Model Were Used for the Baccalaureate, Master's, and Doctorate Programs

	Item	Direct	Rational	Syntactical	Contextual	Inquiry
Practical	60	27	10	0	3	0
Diploma	35	30	15	5	15	0
Associate	35	30	15	7	10	5
*Baccalaureate	15	20	25	15	15	10
*Masters	5	5	15	35	20	20
Doctorate	0	0	5	10	15	70

*Programs that have percentages altered.

the ways illustrated in these tables because they are the programs that would be most affected by new ways of perceiving curriculum.

Using new curriculum-development paradigms, baccalaureate programs would become more focused on the syntactical, an area that relies heavily on student-teacher interaction and that is all but ignored by today's nursing educators. Master's programs would also shift toward more emphasis on the syntactical. It is one of the major purposes of master's programs to prepare clinical specialists, clinical expertise being the focus of syntactical learning. It may be that syntactical learning takes place best in the clinical area or in clinical simulation. Benner's work (1984) certainly verifies that clinical experience is essential and central to it.

Further, the syntactical relies heavily on teacher-student interactions to help students search for and find meanings, view wholes, crystallize insights, evaluate, anticipate, and intuit.

What becomes clear in all of this is that in order to achieve what Botkin, Elmandjra, and Malitza (1979) refer to as "innovative" learning and what the AACN refers to as "professional nursing," one must alter the curriculum in ways to promote teaching that *educates* rather than *trains*. Adding college courses and stressing rationale is insufficient. Socialization through the "hidden curriculum" is insufficient. Syntactical, contextual, and inquiry learning must become legitimate throughout the curriculum.

Alter Our Perception of Teaching and the Role of the Teacher

Sykalys and Watson (1985) reviewed seven studies done in the 1980s: the Paidaia Proposal (1982), Physicians for the 21st Century (1984), President Bok's Report to the Harvard Board of Overseers (1984), The National Institute of Education Report (1984), the National Endowment for Humanities Report (1984), the Institute of Medicine Report (1983), and the National Commission on Nursing Study (1983). From these and the document of the AACN (1986), Sykalys and Watson derived six Curricular Recommendations and five Instructional Recommendations. Those germane to my manifesto are Curricular Recommendations 2 and 4, which read, respectively: "increased emphasis on intellectual skills such as analytic, problem-solving and critical thinking skills" and "increased emphasis on fundamental and essential attitudes and values." These fall into learning types: 4 syntactical, 5 contextual, and 6 inquiry. For Instructional Recommendations, all four recommendations speak to the alteration of our perceptions of teaching and teaching roles. They call for: 1) increased emphasis on "good teaching"; 2) increased emphasis on promoting active modes of learning; 3) increased utilization of Socratic teaching strategies; and 4) increased student-faculty interaction in the learning environment. (See Figure 6.)

Figure 6
The Teachers Roles

Purposes:

1. Insure safety.
2. Provide the climate, the structure, and the dialogue that promotes praxis.

Roles:

1. Design ways to engage the student in mental processes of analysis of cues until patterns are seen that provide paradigms for practice.
2. Raise questions that require reading, observation, analysis, and reflection upon patient care.
3. Nurture the learner.
4. Nurture the ethical ideal.
5. Nurture the caring role.
6. Nurture the creative drive.
7. Nurture curiosity and the search for satisfying ideas.
8. Nurture assertiveness.
9. Support the spirit of inquiry.
10. Nurture the desire to seek dialogue about care and be available for that dialogue.
11. Interact with students as persons of worth, dignity, intelligence, and high scholarly standards.

The message is clear: To mount our revolution we must dispense with the view of the teacher as an information-giver either in the classroom or in the practicum. The teacher's main purpose, beyond the minimal activity of insuring safety, is to provide the climate, the structure, and the dialogue that promotes praxis. The teacher's role is to design ways to engage the student in the mental processes of analysis of cues until patterns are seen that provide paradigms for practice. Further, the teacher's role is to raise questions that require reading, observation, analysis, and reflection upon patient care. The teacher's role is to nurture the learner: to nurture the ethical ideal, to nurture the caring role, to nurture the creative drive, to nurture curiosity and the search for satisfying ideas, to nurture assertiveness and the spirit of inquiry together with the desire to seek dialogue about care, and to be available for that dialogue. The teacher's role is to interact with students as persons of worth, dignity, intelligence, and high scholarly standards.

In the classroom and in practicums, teachers must begin to see themselves as what Stenhouse (1980) calls "expert learners." As expert learners, their primary role revolves around helping students, as novice learners, learn how to learn—how to be scholars—how to think critically—how to gain insights and find meanings—how to see patterns and how to capitalize on their paradigm experiences. Teachers must see their role as structuring learning activities to help achieve these ends.

Essentially, the teacher's main problem is not what to lecture on, nor how to organize that lecture. The teacher's main problems are two: what learning activities to select or design that will promote the type of learning desired and what kinds of teacher-student transactions will best promote educative learning. Solving these two problems must become the central issues in any professional curriculum development paradigm.

To promote educative learning, teachers need a clearer idea of the ways to facilitate syntactical, contextual, and inquiry learning. Some clues can be found in examining learning modalities and heuristics of scholarship. Intellectual modes enable the learner to cope with syntax and inquiry (types 4 and 6) and enable all the other types to make sense to the learner. If teachers recognize the value of these modes, they can raise issues and questions that provide the subject matter for teacher-student interactions. Such interactions would require the student to use these modes in the learning process. In the end, it is

Figure 7
Intellectual Modes That Characterize the Expert Learner

1. Analysis.
2. Critiquing.
3. Recognizing insights.
4. Identifying and evaluating assumptions.
5. Inquiring into the nature of things using all available methods.
6. Projecting, futuring, anticipating, predicting or hypothesizing from knowns to unknowns.
7. Searching for structural or organizational motifs or building them.
8. Engaging in praxis: enabling theory and practice each to inform and shape the other.
9. Evaluating: assessing merit using criteria and expert judgment.
10. Viewing wholes, not just parts in relation to each other.
11. Acknowledging paradigm experiences and cases in ways that enable them to be useful in practice and theorizing.
12. Finding meanings in ideas and experiences.
13. Strategizing.

how well and appropriately the intellectual modes are used that characterizes an expert learner. (See Figure 7.)

Some learners will use these modes in training, but they use them minimally. However, it hardly bears remarking that all learners have insights, find meanings, anticipate, project, and structure. It is the frequency, the habitual approach, the valuing of these intellectual modes, and the expertise of their use that mark educative learning. Further, it is the types of conclusions, ideas, and insights that are derived from these modes that distinguish the educated mind and the quality of abstractions that can be elicited from them by the student.

We Must Change Our Metaphor

The metaphor in nursing education has long been an industrial one wherein schools are seen as some kind of factory and students are referred to as "products." Yet nursing schools are not manufacturers of nurses and graduates are not products. Products are objects, but students, like graduates, are subjects.

Words are powerful things. Speaking of people as products leads to thinking of them as products; thinking of students as products leads to treating them as objects. The behaviorist models of curriculum development are more compatible with the industrial metaphor than is a professional model. For the professional model, I suggest we do not need a metaphor. It is sufficient that we are educators; education has a language, a language of human beings, wherein people who are enrolled are called students and those who fulfill the requirements are called graduates.

We Must Restructure the Relative Roles of the Classroom and the Clinical Practice Area

In practice disciplines, such as nursing, the curriculum plan becomes a lived curriculum within the classroom and clinical practicum. Classroom teaching is often referred to as "theory," but this is a misleading title in that "theory" is encountered in educative teaching regardless of the setting. In professional nursing education, only theory that has an intimate relationship with practice has relevance. Theory that either originates in practice or is tried out (tested) with real people and discussed among nurses and other colleagues can grow, change, develop or become verified . . . in other words, become "living theory." Living theory does not arise in the classroom and then is "tried out" in the practicum. Nor is it the reverse, in which it arises in the practicum and is then discussed to reveal meanings in the classroom. Living theory is encountered in praxis, a dance wherein ideas, concepts, and theories may rise in the intellect from reading, discussions, lectures, classroom learning activities or in practice. Practice both tests and enhances theory, and theory both tests and enhances practice. Each enlightens the other, provoking insights, altering and changing the form, shape, and meanings of each. As the theory evolves, so the practice evolves. In this way, in the truly professional curriculum, each informs the other in the magical whole of praxis.

We Must De-emphasize Curriculum Development and Concentrate on Faculty Development

If faculty have any courses in nursing education at all, they come to us from the Tyler/Bevis legacy. What they know is training, not education. Curriculum development, then, as I said in my introductory remarks, just rearranges things and, if we are lucky, improves on training. In our revolution, all curriculum development starts with faculty development, wherein faculty are helped to make the transition to educational practices, to the art of raising questions that provoke dialogue and facilitate insight, patterns, meanings, and the other characteristics of education discussed earlier. Faculty development must concentrate on helping faculty alter their perception of their role.

If faculty development is successful, the curriculum will change as a natural consequence of faculty dialogue. I will not go into that here, but Joseph Schwab (1979) offers several excellent suggestions about how that process occurs. We must not equate content selection with curriculum development. Content selection is a very small part of the process. Faculty development is the key.

We Must Develop a National Strategy for the Revolution

Without a national strategy, without leadership, there will be lots of talk and little change. Perhaps an evolution that gradually loosens the bondage of institutionalized sanctions supporting the Tyler models may occur, but there will be no great change. We must have a group of leaders to map our strategy, leaders who will give their energy, time, and scholarship to making the revolution a reality. Dreams do come true and we can fly over the rainbow, not from wishing it so but by making it so with commitment and hard work.

CONCLUSION

In conclusion, what is sought for nursing education is a legitimization of the educational and professional elements of curriculum; an

Figure 8
Manifesto for a Curriculum Revolution

Purposes:
1. Substantively change the nature of the graduate of Professional schools.
2. Create a true discipline of nursing.

Recommendations:
1. Deinstitutionalize the Tyler curriculum development model and its mandated products.
2. Make nursing philosophy, research, and education congruent.
3. Distinguish between learning that is training and learning that is educational.
4. Alter perceptions of teaching and the role of the teacher.
5. Abandon the industrial metaphor.
6. Restructure the relative roles of classroom and clinical practice.
7. De-emphasize curriculum development and concentrate on faculty development.
8. Develop a national strategy for curriculum change.

endorsement of the dynamic, creative whole of education; a legitimization of the teaching of inquiry, reflection, criticism, independence, creativity, and caring. It must include all aspects of nursing education, the legitimate, illegitimate, and hidden curricula. A methodology for curriculum development is needed that will provide a new type of graduate, a substantively different graduate, because the planning process emphasizes the selection of experiences and the character and quality of teacher-student interactions instead of closely held, highly structured, prescribed outcomes. The graduate must be different because the values are different, the emphasis placed is different, the roles of teachers and students are different, the types of learning activities are different. In other words, the content may remain similar but the approach to the content is so altered that the curriculum itself is different and consequently the graduates are professionals.

Therefore, it is essential that nursing educators and curriculum experts seek new models for curriculum development that offer a means for developing curriculum that will facilitate students in developing creative, dynamic modes of approaching nursing care. These models must emphasize the selection or creation of learning activities that promote educative learning and teacher-student interactions that help students learn syntax, context, and inquiry.

This can be done only with a different kind of curriculum development: one that provides a wider range of options, a greater scope of ideas, a valuing of active teaching strategies; one that views teacher development as the primary goal and curriculum development as a by-product; one that redefines learning, supports student creative thought as the essence of education, and has an underlying assumption that nursing is a human science.

Eleanor Roosevelt said, "We face the future fortified only with the lessons we have learned from the past. It is today that we must create the world of the future . . . . In a very real sense, tomorrow is now." For nursing education, tomorrow has come.

REFERENCES

American Association of Colleges of Nursing. (1986). *Essentials of College and University Education for Professional Nursing, Final Report*. Washington, DC: Author.

Benner, P. (1984). *From novice to expert: Excellence and power in clinical nursing practice*. Menlo Park, CA: Addison-Wesley Publishing Company.

Bloom, A. (1987) *The closing of the American mind.* New York: Simon and Schuster.

Botkin, J. W., Elmandjra, M., & Malitza, M. (1979). *No limits to learning: Bridging the human gap.* New York: Pergamon Press.

Brown, E. L. (1948). *Nursing for the future.* New York: Russell Sage Foundation.

Chayer, M. (1947). *Nursing in modern society.* New York: G. P. Putnam's Sons.

Dock, L., & Stewart, I. (1920) *A short history of nursing.* New York: G. P. Putnam's Sons.

Eisner, E. (1982). *Cognition and curriculum: A basis for deciding what to teach.* New York: Longman, John Dewey Lecture Series, No. 18.

Eisner, E. (Ed.). (1985). *Learning and teaching the way of knowing, eighty-fourth yearbook of the National Society for the Study of Education, Part II.* Chicago: The University of Chicago Press.

Goldmark, J. (Ed.). (1923). *Study on nursing and nursing education in the United States.* New York: The Rockefeller Foundation.

Kliebard, H. M. (1970). The Tyler rationale. *School Review 78*, 259–272.

Mager, R. (1975). *Preparing instructional objectives* (2 ed.). Belmont, CA: Feron Publishers.

Montag, M. (1951). *The education of nursing technicians.* New York: Putnam.

Munhall, P. L. (1982). Nursing philosophy and nursing research: In apposition or opposition? *Nursing Research, 31*, 176–181.

National League of Nursing Education, Committee on Curriculum. (1917, 1927, 1937). *Curriculum guide for schools of nursing.* New York: National League of Nursing Education.

Nightingale, F. (1867). Suggestions on the subject of providing, training, and organizing nurses for the sick poor in workhouse infirmaries, Appendix No. 3. In L. Seymer (Ed.) (1954). *Selected writings of Florence Nightingale.* New York: Macmillan.

Raths, J. D. (1971). Teaching without specific objectives. *Educational Leadership, 28*, 714–720.

Sakalys, J., & Watson, J. (1985) New directions in higher education: A review of trends. *Journal of Professional Nursing. (1)5*, 293–299.

Sand, O. (1955). *Curriculum study in basic nursing education.* New York: G. P. Putnam's Sons.

Schwab, J. (1979). *Science, curriculum and liberal education: Selected essays.* Chicago: The University of Chicago Press.

Stewart, I. (1947). *The education of nurses, historical foundations and modern trends.* New York: The Macmillan Company.

Stenhouse, L. (Ed.). (1980). *Curriculum research and development in action.* London: Heinemann Educational Books, Ltd.

Taba, H. (1962). *Curriculum development, theory and practice.* New York: Harcourt, Brace and World, Inc.

Tyler, R. W. (1950). *Basic principles of curriculum and instruction*. Chicago: University of Chicago Press.

Watson, J. (1979). *Nursing: The philosophy and science of caring*. Boulder, CO: Colorado Associated University Press.

Watson, J. (1985). *Nursing: Human science and human care: A theory of nursing*. Norwalk, CT: Appleton-Century-Crofts.

Wolf, L. (1947) *Nursing*. New York: Appleton-Century Co., Inc.

BIBLIOGRAPHY

Bevis, E. O. (1982). *Curriculum building in nursing: A process* (3rd ed.). St. Louis: The C. V. Mosby Co.

Bridgman, M. (1953). *Collegiate education for nursing*. New York: Russell Sage Foundation.

Doll, W. E. Jr. (1978). A structural view of curriculum. *Theory into Practice, 17*, 336–348.

Eisner, E. (1985). *The educational imagination, on the design and evaluation of school programs*. New York: Macmillan Publishing Company.

Harmer, B. (1935). *Textbook of the principles and practice of nursing*. New York: The Macmillan Company.

Harmer, B., & Henderson, V. (1955). *Textbook of the principles and practice of nursing*. New York: The Macmillan Company.

Hebert, R. (1981). *Florence Nightingale: Saint, reformer or rebel?* Malabar, FL: Robert E. Krieger Publishing Company.

Pennock, M. (Ed.). (1940). *Makers of nursing history, portraits and pen sketches of one hundred and nine prominent women*. New York: Lakeside Publishing Company.

Roberts, M. (1954). *American nursing, history and interpretation*. New York: The Macmillan Company.

Roby, T. W. (1983, April). *Habits impeding deliberation*. Paper presented at the Annual Meeting of The American Educational Research Association, Montreal, Quebec, Canada.

Schwab, J. (1969). The practical: A language for curriculum. *School Review, 78(11)*, 1–23.

Small, R. (1978). Educational praxis. *Educational Theory. 28*, 214–222.

Stenhouse, L. (1983). *Authority, education and emancipation*. London: Heinemann Educational Books, Ltd.

Woodham-Smith, C. (1951). *Florence Nightingale, 1820–1910*. New York: McGraw-Hill.

4

Curriculum Revolution: An Agenda for Change

Patricia Moccia

The present moment is a particularly important one for us in nursing, as well as for the future of health care in this country. Now seems to be an especially good time for us to come together to think, dream, and plan for the future. As we do so, it may be helpful to remember what Virginia Woolf (1938) wrote half a century ago:

> We are here, on the bridge, to ask ourselves certain questions. And they are very important questions; and we have very little time in which to answer them. The questions that we have to ask and to answer about the procession during this moment of transition are so important that they may well change the lives of all men and women forever. For we have to ask ourselves, here and now, do we wish to join that procession, or don't we? On what terms shall we join that procession? Above all, where is it leading us, the procession of educated men? The moment is short; it may last five years; ten years, or perhaps only a matter of a few months longer. But the questions must be answered; and they are so important that if all the daughters of educated men did nothing, from morning to night, but consider that procession, from every angle, if they did nothing but ponder it and analyze it, and think about it and read about it and pool their thinking and reading, and what they see and what they guess, their time would be better spent than in any other activity now open to them.
>
> . . . Let us never cease from thinking—what is this "civilization" in which we find ourselves? What are these ceremonies and why

> should we take part in them? What are these professions and why should we make money out of them? Where in short is it leading us, the procession of the sons of educated men? (pp. 62–63)

Today, it is all too apparent where the procession of educated men has led. People's lives and well-being are ruptured by economic decisions that serve a company's profit goals at the cost of hundreds and in some cases thousands of jobs. For the good of the corporations, workers are deprived not only of wages but also of their sense of self; their families are deprived of security; and in some cases their children are deprived of food and shelter. Nations spend billions and mortgage future generations so that governments may play the game of one-upmanship and nuclear proliferation, while individuals are left to live and cope with the daily threat of annihilation in the only way they can: through a process of psychic numbing and alienation that eventually infiltrates other parts of their psyche and sabotages their interpersonal relations.

What is worse, all human interactions have been reduced to commodities, to be marketed and bought and sold for profit. The implications of recent public discourse on such issues as surrogate motherhood are astounding. Without apology or embarrassment, life itself has been dissected in legal battles about whether a man who has paid a woman to be artificially inseminated and carry the fetus to term is buying a whole baby or half a baby, since "half the baby is legally his anyway." Contrast this tragic situation with King Solomon's decision (I Kings 3:16) in a much earlier and supposedly less enlightened time.

To many nurses, the day-to-day experience of nursing makes it painfully clear that the procession of educated men has led to ideologies and values that are dominated by what Habermas (1970) refers to as technical-rational-purposive systems of interactions, systems whose goals are the ever more efficient domination and exercise of control over nature and people. As such systems come to dominate all aspects of society, the procession leads further and further away from those systems of interactions whose goals are the preservation, fostering, and nurturing of human potential.

Every day, from moment to moment, nurses witness a society characterized by alienation and dehumanization as they become involved in the lives of the patients who come to their institutions and agencies seeking care, compassion, and help. Every day, they are faced with a growing number of lives that are increasingly fragmented, constricted, and impoverished as a result of public and social policies. At first glance, these policies seem to have little to do with health care. On closer examination, however, we see that nurses' work experiences are filled with firsthand accounts of the impact of national and state policies on the lives of individuals, families, groups, children, mothers, the elderly, and minority communities. The effects of social ideologies that value technical-rational interests rather than human concerns and interests have infiltrated patients' lives. As a result, we have begun to experience for ourselves the consequences of a society that refuses to value caring: our work is increasingly fragmented, deskilled and pressured, and our contributions are increasingly undervalued or even completely unacknowledged.

The problem facing all concerned with health care and the health of society and civilization is that the expertise and skills necessary to reform the health care system and to promote a healthier society already exist within nursing's common body of knowledge, but they are in danger of being lost unless the profession's crisis of numbers is resolved. At the same time, because the profession's crisis reflects those in the larger system, its resolution depends on changes in that system—changes that, in turn, depend on nursing's particular expertise, that is, the expertise and knowledge that nurses have created and shared with each other as they have gone about the daily work of caring for people within the current systems, ensuring that people are cared for, and developing and administering systems that support caregivers. Without nurses and nursing knowledge, society and the health care system will lose the knowledge of how to care for people despite social structures and systems that would argue against caring encounters.

What, then, is to be done about such a civilization and such a system?

CHOICES FACING NURSING

There are many avenues through which we can create social change and many choices open to us as we decide whether to join the procession of educated men. The general choice facing us as leaders in nursing and nursing education has been clearly stated by MIT Professor Donald Schon (1987):

> In the varied topography of professional practice, there is a high, hard ground overlooking a swamp. On the high ground, manageable problems lend themselves to solution through the application of research-based theory and technique. In the swampy lowland,

> messy, confusing problems defy technical solution. The irony of this situation is that the problems of the high ground tend to be relatively unimportant to individuals or society at large, however great their technical interests might be, while in the swamp lie the problems of greatest human concern.
>
> The practitioner must choose. Shall he remain on the high ground where he can solve relatively unimportant problems according to prevailing standards of rigor, or shall he descend to the swamp of important problems and nonrigorous inquiry? (p. 3)

We are all acutely aware of the enormous difficulties that nurse educators have faced as they fought to establish nursing as a distinct and legitimate part of the university and nurse educators as unique and valuable members of the academic community. Each of us owes a tremendous personal and professional debt to those who, like the faculty here, were part of these accomplishments. Undoubtedly we will face additional battles as we continue to challenge the social forces and societal structures that would keep women from defining their worlds and nurses from thinking about people and their health. Still, I believe, nursing education and nurse educators have by and large achieved legitimacy.

We must, however, continue to ask ourselves what we mean by nursing education. If nursing education is only about securing positions of influence for nursing and for individual nurses, we already have what we want. We can stop, enjoy our justly won desserts, and simply continue as we have until now. But if nursing education is also about creating and sharing the knowledge that will be useful to people as they strive to develop, create, and fulfill their potential to live healthy and productive lives, there is still much to be done.

To me, as to many others, there seem to be some indications—notably our painstaking attention to acceptable curricula and our seeming obsession with course and terminal objectives—that the acceptance of nursing into the academic community may have come at too high a price for the profession, nurse educators, their students, and the people who look to nurses for care to pay. In order to be accepted in research-driven universities or technically driven colleges, we may have given up much of the humanity and caring that identify nurses as nurses and nursing as nursing.

If this is the case, the major challenge facing nursing education is how to reclaim whatever we may have lost in our quest for legitimacy before it is irretrievable. How can we move our focus away from the particular behaviors or characteristics of our students and back to an understanding of them as whole beings? How can we relearn how to respect their humanity and dignity rather than their isolated rationality? How can we reintroduce feelings, emotion, and imagination into the shared spaces between teacher and student and between nurse and patient? In short, how can we remake education as an activity that affirms and encourages the humanity of all involved? Now that nursing has attained a position of influence in the academic community, it must use that position to change the nature of the academic community.

"THE PERSONAL IS POLITICAL"

How can we accomplish the necessary changes? According to one school of thought, we must change the world. According to another, we must change our innermost lives. Although at first glance these two approaches to change may appear to be in opposition, they are actually complementary. The dialectical relationship between them has incredible potential for creating change if we remember that, as the feminists of the 1960s said, "the personal is political."

My aim in this paper is twofold: (1) to formulate a strategic agenda for the curriculum revolution that has been called for and (2) to suggest ways in which organized nursing can rise to the challenge of such a revolution. Accordingly, I propose three goals, which I will discuss in more detail below. The first goal is political, the second is personal, and the third is concerned with the relationship between these two aspects of our lives:

1. To work to abolish the fee-for-service, profit-driven health care system;
2. To reform the accreditation process by drawing it away from its fixation on structures and their administration and toward a concern with process and the personal relationships between teachers and students; and
3. To attempt to create a "web of consciousness" among nurses that will allow us to articulate a shared vision of what a healthy society might look like.

Abolition of Fee-For-Service

Organization of the health care system on a fee-for-service basis has implications for nursing and for nursing education. The procession of educated men has led us to a profit-driven biomedical enterprise that now finds itself without the expertise or skills necessary to meet the health care needs of a population that is increasingly aged, chronically ill, and without access to health services.

There are several significant problems with this approach to structuring health care. First, sicker patients will continue to suffer, since it is more profitable to the provider to serve healthier patients who need less service. Second, the more than 40 million Americans who have no insurance simply will get no care. Third, a profit-driven fee-for-service system is unable to exert sufficient control over costs, because as long as providers control the number of services in order to increase their profits, the aggregate costs to the payors in the health care system will continue to be difficult to control. Finally, and perhaps most profoundly, the process of determining and attaching a fee for service necessarily distorts the humanity of both providers and patients. When the health care system attempts to isolate services and fees, people's complex health needs are separated into discrete units, by design. This separation, which is necessitated by the fee-for-service approach, is untrue to the reality of the patient's experience. In addition, since life and death are subject to the same market conditions that any commodity is, people are reduced to object status, and interpersonal relations become avenues of commerce. As a result, the isolation and dehumanization of the larger society is reinforced and sustained by the health care system.

Consequently, though fee-for-service is seemingly a financial and economic issue, the choice between it and some other form of reimbursement is actually a choice to reinforce and legitimize one understanding of human phenomena rather than another and to adopt one philosophy of interpersonal relations rather than another. As such, the choice between fee-for-service and some other form of reimbursement has significant implications for curricula and pedagogy—that is, what we teach and how we teach it.

Reform of Accreditation

Nurse educators, like most educators, love to think of education as a progressive process that liberates people and opens new opportunities for them. In light of the critiques of the past 20 years, however, it is impossible not to question that trusting view. Various analyses have presented an alternate view of education as a conservative force that perpetuates the status quo by extending the social discrimination of contemporary society into future generations (Apple, 1985). For example, the philosopher Maxine Greene (1986) reaches a disquieting conclusion about where the procession of educated men has led, as she speaks of individual graduates: "There is little sense of agency even among the brightly successful; there is little capacity to look at things as if they could be otherwise" (p. 438). If education's promise has been compromised into its very contradiction, how has this happened?

Greene (1986), citing Marcuse, reminds us that we are perhaps more than anything else an administered society. I believe that nursing education, like many other educational fields, focuses on its administration—that is, on its technical aspects—at the expense of the lived experience of students and teachers. Because of the current accreditation process, we are obsessed with content and with measurable objectives. We live and breathe these things: we create and re-create them, we design courses and lectures according to them, we write reports about them, we are evaluated by them, and our accreditation depends on them.

Many years ago, we faced the choice between the high ground and the swamp. We chose the high ground: we went for programs that were logically organized, well administered, and open to technical measures and manipulation. At that time, we had no choice; we needed to establish our norms. Now, however, it is time for us to turn back to the swamp of interpersonal relations between student and teacher. It is time to focus on the process of education—the student-teacher relationship—rather than on its content or anything else.

The educator Ira Shor (1986) argues for a critical pedagogy that is participatory, research-minded, critical, values-oriented, multicultural, student-centered, experimental, and interdisciplinary. It is this kind of relationship that we must seek to create with our students, and it is to the degree that we create such a relationship that we should be accredited. Only this kind of relationship can give us the power to change the world and our innermost selves.

The NLN should be commended for its decision to reissue a classic work, *Humanistic Nursing* (Paterson & Zderad, 1988). In this book, the authors, drawing on the transcendental philosopher Martin Buber, locate the source of the power embedded in an interpersonal exchange, where the call of one person is shared with the potential response of another: When the potential response becomes real, an incredible amount of power is generated. There is the power of the participants to change and become more than they were before the exchange; and there is the power of the participants to transcend the situation by engaging the events whirling around them and together trying to make sense of their worlds and find a meaning to their existence.

When the call and response between two people is as honest as it can be, there is the revolutionary power of which the poet Muriel Rukeyser speaks: "What would happen if one woman told the truth about her life?/The world would split open" (Greene, 1986, p. 429). It is this same authenticity that we search for in our friendships and with our lovers. We look for relationships with people who really listen to what we are saying, who really try to understand our lived experiences of the world, and who ask the same from us. Finding such relationships brings us an intense and exhilarating feeling of self-affirmation and a comforting sense of well-being.

If, as holistic beings, we are the implicate order explicating itself, as Bohm (1983) and Newman (1987) suggest, then the responsibilities of those of us who wish to help (such as nurses) and those of us who wish to nurture (such as educators) include making sense out of the chaos into which we have been led by the procession of educated men. When we help students or patients to make sense of their realities by bringing meaning to them, we make sense of and bring meaning to our own realities. And when we help create meaning, it is easier for us to remember why we chose nursing or nursing education and why we continue to choose it despite what a lousy, underpaid, and undervalued job it has become in today's marketplace. When we get past our science and theories, our technical prowess, and our titles and positions of influence, it is the shared moment of authenticity—whether between nurse and patient or between student and teacher—that makes us take heart and allows us to move forward with our own life projects. The same is true for deans of schools of nursing, administrators of delivery systems, the executives and staff of nursing and professional organizations, or colleagues on a research project. It is the authentic dialogue between people that makes any activity worthwhile, regardless of whether or not it is called successful by others.

Perhaps this reissue of a classic work will help to remind us of another way of developing our power. Perhaps we can once again look for and call for authentic dialogue with our patients, our students, and our colleagues. The method outlined by Paterson and Zderad (1988) is clear and direct: discuss, question, convey, clarify, argue, and reflect. Implicit in this method is the assumption that whereas each one of us is unique, we all need to be and to do with each other if we are to grow. Also implicit is a celebration of the power of our choices.

If the NLN or any organization wants to accredit schools, it should make sure that it is asking the really important question ers model caring behavior? Are there structured opp meaningful dialogue and practice? Is the humanity of and teachers affirmed by their interactions? Do the stud stand themselves to be social-cultural beings? Do they share ...se of community and collegiality with their teachers? With other students? With nurses?

In fact, I suggest that the whole accreditation process can be reduced to two simple questions (adapted from Nell Noddings, 1986 and the work of Jean Watson, 1988). As the reviewers examine the school's philosophy, its conceptual framework, its library resources, and whatever else seems important to them they need only ask:

1. What effect does it all have on the person being taught and the person teaching?
2. What effect will it have on the caring community we are trying to build?

Creation of a "Web of Consciousness"

A recent work by William Drake (1987), *The First Wave*, raises several interesting points that we should consider as we face the challenges of today and the choices before us. The book is about 27 American women poets—including such artists as Amy Lowell, Marianne Moore, Sara Teasdale, and Anne Spencer—who between 1915 and 1945 approached their work not as heroic and isolated individuals but rather as a community of artists who nurtured and mentored and inspired each other to creativity.

These women faced two choices as they sought a space within which to be creative and to do their work. They could either (1) accept a defensive position and work within the limits of power laid down by others (in their case, male poets; in our case, the biomedical profit-driven enterprise) or (2) find a new empowerment through a new vision (in their case, a women-centered vision; in our case, a nurse-centered vision). The women poets made several key discoveries: (1) a "web of consciousness" was essential to their creative growth and survival; (2) the power to be and the power to create in the face of discouragement has its source in love, in a passionate involvement that releases the power of its participants to become their fully human selves; and (3) despite their great intimacy, empowering friendships need not be exclusive or limited. In other words, they found that they needed community as well as personal connection.

Now more than ever, we need to create and articulate our own visions. In 1950 Isabel Maitland Stewart (1984), who was head of Teachers College Division of Nursing for many years, remarked:

> Among those who have led nursing movements of the past were a number of great spiritual leaders who lifted nursing to a high spiritual plane and made it a vital part of the movement for human welfare and the advancement of civilization. (p. 381)

We need such leaders now to revive the spirit of nursing, to unite the whole body of nurses in a common purpose, and to give us a new vision of our part in the world of the future.

What is this vision? What will it look like? How can we ever hope to create a common vision when we cannot even decide on something as minor—compared with the profound experiences of life, death, passion, and desire—as entry into practice?

One way of beginning to answer these questions is to follow Greene's (1980) suggestion:

> Perhaps we might begin by releasing our imaginations and summoning up the traditions of freedom in which most of us were reared. We might try to make audible again the recurrent themes for justice and equality. We might reactivate the resistance to materialism and conformity. (p. 440)

Another is to join forces with organizations like Nurses for Progressive Social Change, who have formulated an agenda for the coming campaign year that includes attempting to convince the political candidates of the following points:

- that adequate housing is necessary for health;
- that adequate nutrition is necessary for health;
- that meaningful employment is necessary for health;
- that nuclear disarmament is necessary for health;
- that the end to domination—of individuals, peoples, nations, and nature—is necessary for health; and
- that access to just and humane health service must be assured for all individuals, irrespective of their ability to pay, social category, prior health status, or place of residence.

CONCLUSIONS

We are faced with many choices as we decide whether to join the procession of educated men and how to choose between the high ground or the swamp. Should we adopt the values of commerce and redesign health care systems accordingly? Should we accept competition as the modus operandi or insist on other measures for people in need? How do we decide who will be cared for and who will not? Who will pay and how much?

As Greene (1986) reminds us, "These are dark and shadowed times, and we need to live them, standing before one another, open to the world." Perhaps it is time for us to turn away from the exchange between buyers and sellers, providers and consumers, and turn back to an exchange between two people trying to understand the space they share. Perhaps it is time for us to enter into dialogue with patients, since they are the ones most affected by these questions. Perhaps it is time for us to hear their call and respond authentically; perhaps it is time they were permitted to hear ours. And perhaps it is time to teach our students this.

I believe it is time, for many reasons, but mainly because, as Paterson and Zderad (1988) argue, only then will our lived experiences in health care and education have any real meaning. Only when we grant love, passion, feeling, and imagination the same legitimacy that we grant reason, logic, and techniques; only when we restore our sense of community and reclaim our place as active participants in our world; only then will we be healthy as individuals, a profession, and a world community.

Now that we know what to do intellectually, we must commit our love and our passions to doing it.

REFERENCES

Apple, M. W. (1985). *Education and power*. Boston: Ark Paperbacks.

Bohm, D. (1983). *Wholeness and the implicate order*. London: Ark Paperbacks.

Drake, W. (1987). *The first wave*. New York: Macmillan.

Greene, M. (1986). In search of a critical pedagogy. *Harvard Educational Review, 56*(4), 427–441.

Habermas, J. (1970). *Toward a rational society* (J. Shapiro, Trans.). Boston: Beacon Press.

Newman, M. (1987). *Health as expanding consciousness.* St. Louis: C.V. Mosby Co.

Noddings, N. (1986). Fidelity in teaching, teacher education, and research for teaching. *Harvard Educational Review, 56*(4), 496–510.

Paterson, J. & Zderad, L. (1988). *Humanistic nursing.* New York: National League For Nursing.

Schon, D. A. (1987). *Educating the reflective practitioner.* San Francisco: Jossey-Bass.

Shor, I. (1986). Equality is excellence: Transforming teacher education and the learning process. *Harvard Educational Review, 56*(4), 406–426.

Stewart, I. M. (1984). *The education of nurses.* New York: Garland. (Original work published 1950)

Watson, J. (1988) *Nursing: Human science and human care.* New York: The National League for Nursing.

Woolf, V. (1960). *Three guineas.* San Diego: Harcourt Brace Jovanovich. (Original work published 1938)

5

Phenomenology: A Foundation for Nursing Curriculum

Carolyn Oiler Boyd

INTRODUCTION

Phenomenological philosophy is a relatively new source of inspiration for nursing. Paterson and Zderad (1976) are the first nurses to interpret phenomenology in nursing in a formal way, in their metatheoretical essays in *Humanistic Nursing*. Another interpretation is found in Parse's (1981) *Man-Living-Health*. Others (Munhall & Oiler, 1986; Oiler, 1982, 1986; Omery, 1983; Ray, 1985) have interpreted phenomenology in nursing research. And still others have indicated an interest in the potential of phenomenology as a method for developing nursing knowledge, if not an explicit commitment to it (Benner, 1983; Watson, 1985). Certainly, the word "phenomenology" has gained our attention, and we find it used to refer to an attitude, an orientation, a research method, a philosophy, and a school of thought. It is all of these. It is not surprising or undesirable that nurse interpreters of phenomenology have different inspirations, but it is confusing to anyone hoping to learn about phenomenology from them. I begin this discussion, then, not with a promise to clarify this situation, but with an acknowledgment that I am but an interpreter; and one who is very much still in the process of coming to understand phenomenology. One still incomplete sense that I have about phenomenology is this: it invites—even requires—laying claim to it for interpretation. In this sense, there is no right or wrong understanding of it; there are only individual possessions of it.

Generally, such theorists and phenomenologically-linked thinkers as Paterson and Zderad (1976), Parse (1981), Watson (1985), Benner (1983), and our growing league of qualitative researchers have expressed an interest in nursing as a social and interpersonal impetus for attestation of humanness. They have located support for this interest in phenomenological and existential philosophy. Their works are rebellions against social and health care forces that impose on us and threaten individual freedom, choice, and becoming. We can trace their rebellions to the grounding provided in our humanistic heritage and in their study of humanistic philosophers, social scientists, and artists. It is not difficult to trace in our own literature (Orlando, 1961; Ujhely, 1968; Wiedenbach, 1965) calls to attend to the human exchanges in nursing, to subjectivity, to experiential phenomena, and to humanistic aims. Yet, this current is not dominant; it has not provided overriding guidance to our curricula, nursing practice, or to our research. Instead, we stand vulnerably in the wake of a spiraling system of controls on human irregularity made possible by "scientific progress." For some of us, the human condition—what it means to exist, to be alive in a world seized by technology—is an appropriate, even important focus for nursing. Existentialism and phenomenology provide a lens.

Existential themes were interpreted in nursing situations in the literature of the 1960s; phenomenology, in the literature of the late 1970s. Why have these sources of inspiration failed to provide us with more? What contains their influence? First, there is a problem with language. Anyone who has read phenomenologically-inspired nursing literature knows that such terms as *intentionality, essence*, and *being-in-the-world* are baffling and foreign to our customary vocabulary. Further, the terms refer to concepts that feature ambiguity, convolution, and paradox. Phenomenology takes us not only into a world of new words, but also into radically different ways of thinking. We are thrust from a relative security with the orderliness of systems into ideas and a perspective that scorn definition, procedure, determination, and abstractions. Beyond these obstacles, we are uncertain as to what difference a struggle with complexity will make for us. Also, there are competing interests and hopes, if not convictions, that scientific prescriptions will resolve our concerns. Assertiveness training, time management, stress management and the like preoccupy us. New theories proliferate, gain popularity, and become curriculum requirements. We are bursting at the seams.

Yet, the interest in humanism, in feminism, in qualitative paradigms survives; and, in recent years, has culminated in a new level of scholarship in our work. Despite science and scientific progress, people continue to suffer. Some argue that suffering is intensified. Our tensions and unease prompt us to look beyond science for a sense of balance.

In this paper, I will indicate general implications of phenomenological philosophy for nursing curricula. In the spirit of the conference's revolutionary theme, I will proceed without concern for integration, compromise, or accommodation of phenomenological ideas with extant curricular orientations, but believe that this needs to be addressed; that is, how can a phenomenological perspective be blended or coexist with other curricula perspectives so that the strengths of all perspectives are preserved?

CENTRAL PHENOMENOLOGICAL CONCEPTS/THEMES

Before offering interpretations for nursing curricula, I will briefly describe central phenomenological themes and concepts.

Collectively, these themes provide an open framework descriptive of the nature of being human: the first distinguishing feature of the phenomenological perspective. Rather than starting with a philosophy and constructing a curriculum, phenomenology grounds us only in an understanding of the nature of being human. There are fewer linear, derived guidelines and prescriptives, more openness, and more constancy in processes of choice. A curriculum philosophy—as a set of statements descriptive of beliefs and values about people, health, nursing, society, learning, and teaching—is constantly chosen and created from a phenomenological foundation that directs us to examine and *confront ourselves* in our nursing, our teaching, and our learning. A phenomenological perspective is antithetical to a curriculum process that establishes fixed patterns to be imposed on the particularities of students and teachers.

Figure 1 summarizes the relationship among phenomenological concepts or themes under consideration: consciousness and embodiment, experience and perception. Consciousness is life itself; it is existing in the world through the relations of bodily systems. Merleau-Ponty (1962) states:

> "The world is not what I think but what I live through."
>
> (p. xvii)

Figure 1
Central Concepts

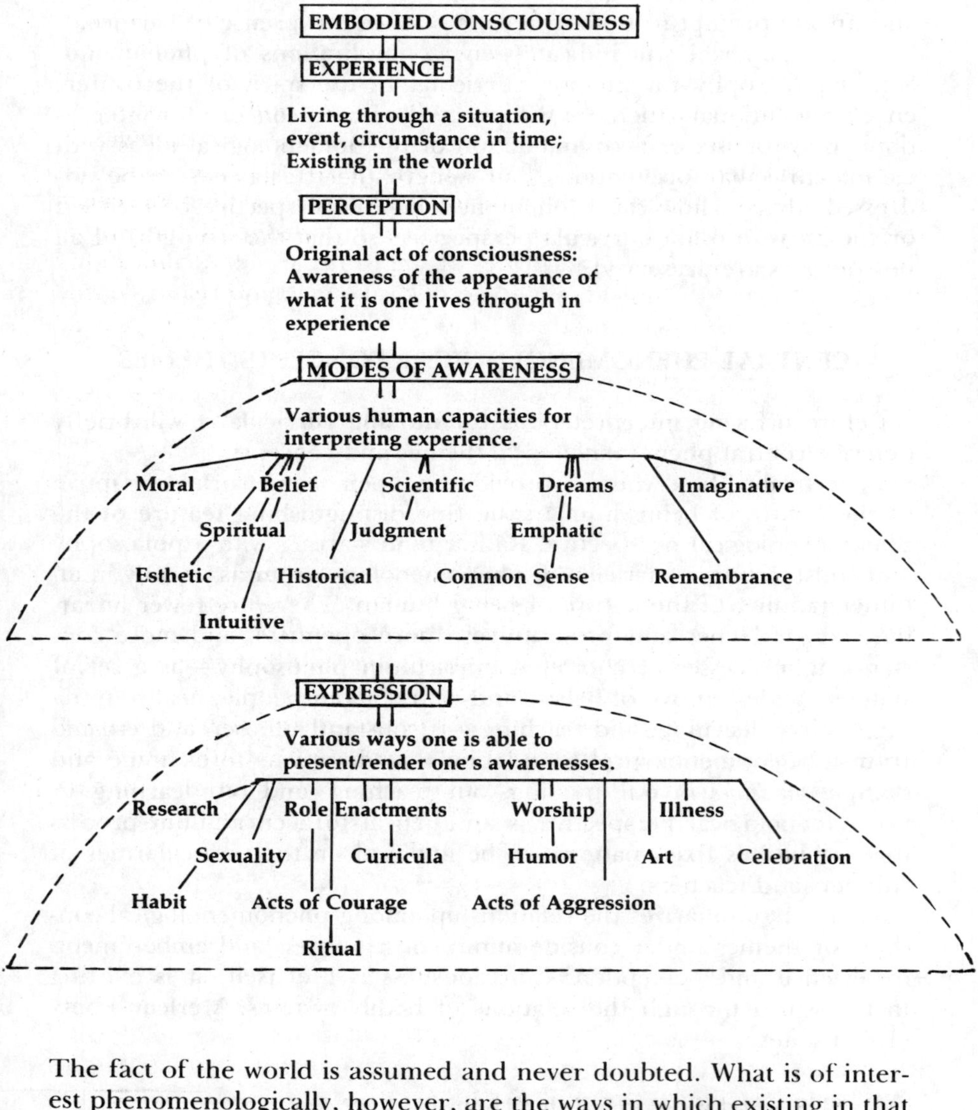

The fact of the world is assumed and never doubted. What is of interest phenomenologically, however, are the ways in which existing in that world is possible. Phenomenology recognizes consciousness as simultaneous contact with the world and with oneself. One is always conscious of something. The world comes to be for the individual in his or her engagement with it. The idea of a subjective and objective world is eliminated. Instead, the phenomenological view of reality is holistic; reality is a subjective presence in a world.

Embodiment refers to the individual's body as his or her natural access to the world, producing what Merleau-Ponty (1962) calls one's "gaze" (p. 67). This means that consciousness is expressed in a particular manner of approach to the world; and the approach (gaze) is brought into being by one's bodily existence in the world. Bodily assuming a position in the world, or being caught up in it, determines the horizon-object structure for the individual. In this sense, human reality is perspectival. Biography, past experience, knowledge of the world, and the social and political facticities of the world are all qualifications of gaze. In this way, individual perspective is formed and reality constituted. Schutz (1970) defines this further:

> The origin of all reality is subjective, whatever excites and stimulates our interest is real. To call a thing real means that this thing stands in a certain relation to ourselves. (p. 207)

Lived experience is the focus of attention in phenomenology. Experience is not what we think, but what we live through. It is existing in a world; and, in the phenomenological sense, communicates the indivisible experiencing subject and experienced object. Perception, the original act of consciousness, refers to the awareness of the appearances of things. The world is not created by the subject's involvement with it, but it is discovered through perception.

For Merleau-Ponty, the world is not perceived through a combination of sensations and perspectives. Rather, relation with the world is a living impulse; coherence in the world is lived. Perception provides access to experience of the world as it is given prior to any analysis we might make of it. As Merleau-Ponty (1962) has stated, "To perceive is to render oneself present to something through the body" (p. 42). The world as perceived, then, is the first reality.

The perceived world, in the phenomenological view, is distinct from the scientific explanation of perception as an act of consciousness, like deciding or reasoning. Rather, the perceived world is a totality in which relations are comprised and organized. It is a totality open to an infinite variety of perspectives, merging, for each individual, into a unique lived style. Perception presents us with evidence of the world not as it is thought, but as it is lived.

Based on experience and perception, other human capacities for awareness enable us to bring meaning to our lives and world. (See Figure 1.) Scientific awareness is one mode for interpreting experience that we strive to develop in nursing education. However, in the phenomenological view, scientific awareness is one *possible* perspective. Like other modes of awareness, it posits what is to be figure; what, ground. In so doing, it provides a particular way of looking at things, and yields a particular interpretation of reality. In phenomenology, science is a second-order reality that takes its proper place among other interpretive modes of awareness.

Finally, such phenomena as research, art, and humor are seen as significant expressions available to human beings; they are ways to present or render awareness. They are consequences, in a sense, of the ways in which we make sense of our existence; sensible outcomes of perspectives taken up in the world.

In this cursory overview of a complex and paradoxical philosophy, my essential point is this: our knowledges about the world are constructed on human experience and within a world of others, objects, and events. Multiple realities are possible because there are multiple capacities for awareness and expression. Phenomenology is quintessentially a human interest that focuses on ways of existing in a world. It is concerned not with the "truth" of the world, but with the realities possible through human involvement with it. Table 1 provides a summary of the central thematic statements in this discussion.

In phenomenology, the aim is to recover original perception. It in-

Table 1
Central Themes

To exist is to exist in a world.
Consciousness is always consciousness *of something*.
One is bodily situated in the world in a particular way, and thus one is tied to it in a perspective. One exists and is conscious through a concrete bodily involvement in the world.
Experience refers to living through a situation, event or circumstance in time. It can only be known reflectively.
Perception, the original act of consciousness, is awareness of the *appearance* of phenomena in experience, and is constituted in one's perspective.
Various modes of awareness (acts of consciousness) characterize human capability. Built on perception, they provide various ways of interpreting (constituting meaning in) experience. Awareness in a particular mode is a matter of taking up a perspective on experience.
The range of human expression, ways to present one's awareness, strengthens our links to the world through bodily involvement with things, others, and ourselves.

volves expanding awareness, becoming wide-awake. It involves coming to know about choices, about self-creation through choices. It also involves discomfort over the knowledge of individual freedom and responsibility.

To be alive in the fullest sense, from the phenomenological point of view, is to be fully aware and thereby capable of responsible choosing. This is the assumed value in phenomenology. If accepted as a point of departure, phenomenology directs us to processes rather than prescriptions—becoming aware, choosing, and acting are thus all valued rather than adhering to selected concepts of health, for example, or applying some set of procedures to a problem.

The idea of existence as an embodied consciousness intending toward a world of things and others eliminates traditional conceptions of subjective and objective. For any given person, existence is involvement in a world. We are drawn by this way of thinking about the nature of being human to a recognition of the centrality of context, interpersonal relations, and multidimensional truths. I can know the world only through my bodily involvement with it. This way of my knowing is individual and unique, yet it could not come to be except through my engagements in the world. The fixities of nursing—its history, its requirements, its culture—did not determine me, make me the nurse I am, give me my perspective, engulf me in a ready-made external reality. Nursing has been constituted in my intending toward it.

Another theme central to phenomenology is that experience refers to living through events, situations, or circumstances. It becomes "known" to us after the fact when we reflect on it. To "know" an experience directly and immediately is not strictly possible. As we turn back to see it, we are now in a new experience of reflecting on an experience that has just passed. In other words, *knowing* what one is living through is interpreted experience and the best we can do is to be aware of our awarenesses; to recognize that knowledge is interpreted reality. Such self-consciousness serves to expand awareness, confront us with our freedom, and point us toward the necessity of choice and action. Reflection, self-awareness, and responsibility, then, are all strategic concepts to carry forward into nursing curricula if education is envisioned as a facilitator of human development and becoming.

The significance of phenomenology for nursing resides in its refusal to accede to a world that is already given in objectivity. It is you who constitute the world. You do not *create* it, but it is you who experience it and give it meaning. You bring values into being through the meanings you attach to objectives, events, or circumstances. It is you who

Table 2
Perceived and Interpreted Experience

Experience & Perception	Interpreted Experience
1st Reality	2nd Order Realities
• having a mastectomy	• concepts of loss, grieving, body image
• being old	• infantalization
• living through a divorce	• anticipatory problem solving
• learning to use crutches	• self-care

establish what is figure, what is ground, thereby bringing order out of chaos in the world. Phenomenology embraces all of this; it is restless, desirous, expectant, rebellious, and interrogative in its recognition of the gaps between what is given and what is to be through human perspective, choice, and action. What better way is there to approach our educational mission than to recognize and use human powers to perceive anew, to orient ourselves in the world through choices, to *construct* our own world?

Table 2 contrasts perceived experience with the interpreted experience rendered by our theories, concepts, and role sets. The first or original realities of having a mastectomy, being an old person, living through a divorce, and learning to use crutches refer to living through events and circumstances in relation to a world of others, objects, and contexts. Such concepts as loss, grieving, infantalization, and self-care provide us with a way of interpreting these experiences. They comment on experience, and vary in how satisfyingly they adhere to the experiences themselves in their complexity. Our knowledge of role and consequent role enactments, such as anticipatory problem solving or self-care goal setting, also impose an order and meaning on the experience. These examples are intended to draw attention to how automatically we use the scientific perspective, assigning our knowledges truth-values without necessarily scrutinizing their "fit" with experience and often without profiting from other perspectives available to us.

IMPLICATIONS FOR NURSING

This overview of a phenomenological foundation of concepts and themes will take on added clarity as the discussion explores the perspective phenomenology lends to selected nursing concerns. I will describe a common dilemma—performing a professional role and being a person—and indicate how the phenomenological concept of coexistence in experience helps to resolve that tension. Various modes of awareness will be noted as positions or perspectives one can assume to look at and know about in lived experiences in nursing. The point I wish to make is this: coexisting with a patient, being engaged with him or her in experience, is not a problem. It is the perspective, the awareness of the experience that can be problematic, create tension, mislead, and burn us out. Expanded awareness, multiplicity in perspectives, will be promoted as the preferred way to construct a nursing perspective, the preferred way to use nursing as a self-actualizing project.

The Role and Person of Nurse

Helping behaviors and professional codes coincide in the conceptual developments of the idea of a nurse's self. The significance of "nurse as person" is usually reduced to selected biographical characteristics (e.g., age and socioeconomic background) that are seen to influence the nurse's ability to help a patient in any given situation. Viewed as potential barriers to helping behaviors and to effectiveness in the helping process, the nurse's person is conceptualized almost as if these identifying features were a nuisance in the professional's work arena. Generally, personal involvement of the nurse has been regarded as antithetical to the features and qualities of the helping role.

Since its emergence from the nursing literature of the 1950s, concern with the therapeutic use of self has become firmly rooted in nursing's way of thinking. Although the once sacrosanct one-to-one relationship in nursing has given way to group, family, and community orientations, the tenets of therapeutic use of self continue to apply and to remain prominent in nursing curricula, practice ideals, and research foci. Increasingly, nurses are instructed in the art of nursing through theoretical models which guide the nurse to practice the behaviors of a professional demeanor. Through a socializing process, concepts are used to transform the nurse-patient experience so that students learn to be professional. Empathy becomes technique; the individual, an object; holism, a multifaceted approach; and humanism, a professional commodity. As human factors are professionalized in this way, a gap between role and person is created. Nurses can and do become estranged from the person that enacts the role. Student nurses tend to lose their natural access to themselves as an outcome of professional role requirements and the conflict between scientifically objective role and humanly involved person.

The conflict between nurse person and nurse role is an acknowledged fact. It is seen as the nurse's vulnerability to emotional exhaustion and her defensive patterns established against it. Scientific objectivity is seen by some as a solution to this conflict. For the nurse, it can be used as a protection against the depletion of personal energy that accrues from being closely involved in the patient's situation. Knowing the patient's situation through his or her perspective is explained as an essentially cognitive process in which the nurse has control over the meaning the patient's situation has for her.

Some authors stress the functional importance and necessity of role. In this view, scientific objectivity is unequivocally valued over other modes of awareness and understanding. But, in this resolution of the tension between person and role, does personal involvement continue unabated? Is it really possible to eliminate emotional involvement, or is it a matter of defending against it by driving it underground?

An example from nursing may clarify this argument, and is presented schematically in Figure 2 to indicate how experience becomes layered over with conceptualizations and interpretations. In caring for

Figure 2
An Example of Sedimentation and Choice

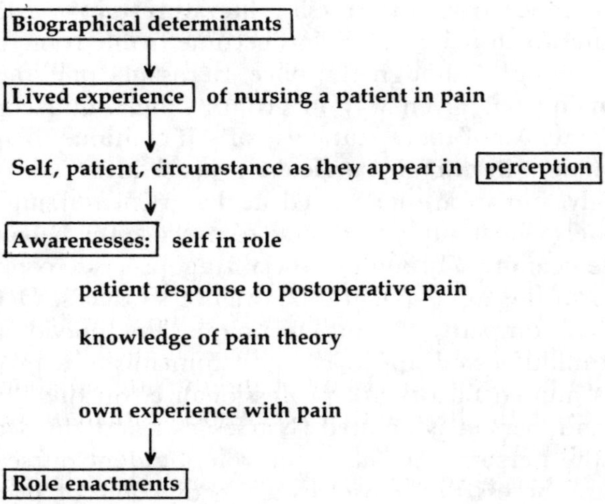

a surgical patient with pain, the nurse is situated in the experience by virtue of a variety of biographical determinants—her age, ethnic identity, cultural beliefs, and so on. She is further situated by such influences as her learned role and past experiences. In living through the experience of nursing her patient, these factors all come to bear, yet do not determine the experience in a cause-effect fashion. There is a singular quality to each experience that relates to possibility, freedom within the limits of time, and choice. The experience the nurse lives through with the patient is contingent also on the patient's influences and possibilities. The nurse's self, the patient, their shared circumstance, and the nursing experience appear in perception and are interpreted through the nurse's modes of awareness, such as objective awareness of self performing a role, scientific awareness of the patient's behavioral response to pain, and perhaps reflective awareness of one's own experience with pain. The nurse might also attend to her empathic and intuitive awareness, but if primarily attuned to her knowledge of pain theory, for example, and to other ways of scientific appraisal in the situation, her expressions will be concerned with such role enactments as structured pain assessment and performance of pain management protocols. It is obvious that exploitation of multiple awareness is desirable.

The tension between nurse as person and nurse as professional role is experienced when we think about it. In experience one is involved as a person through one's role. Without this intending toward the world in the role of nurse, there would not be this nursing experience, but some other.

What does this mean for nursing in its notion of itself as social, interpersonal in nature, and in its aim to help? Nurses are, in the nursing situation, involved with their clients who form, in part, the social world in which nurses exist. Nursing existence is, paradoxically and ambiguously, both the reality constituted by the nurse and the phenomenal field wherein it can occur. In other words, the nurse both creates and is created by the world. In the phenomenological view, the person and the world choose each other.

The nurse's role, her professional self, and the nurse as person in the social world are *not* separate dimensions of the same reality. The elements of role and person can be listed and examined as separate entities, but they do not *cause* the reality of the nursing situation. Rather, they are collectively the history that is the social situation we are concerned with in nursing.

As we think of existence as being-in-the-world, the relation of nurse and patient is a coming together of each of their experiences from the same situation they share. We are so tied to the world that the others in it are central to our own existence. In other words, individual existence is, in Merleau-Ponty's term, a "coexistence."

The nurse and patient are in a primary relation of existing together in the world. More fundamentally, they are tied in a relation which is prior to the nurse or the patient objectifying each other. When the nurse turns away from the relation, she can think about herself separately as person and as nurse. In the same way, she can turn from the relation in experience and think about the patient as a person, role or object of her care. It is when we choose to turn away from the relation and place it as an object in thought that the problem of being therapeutic arises. Objectified, the coexistence of nurse and patient in experience seems to be understandable only by summoning the parts of participants to analysis.

Attempts to understand the nurse-patient relationship and to identify ways of being that are therapeutic for another must be directed to the relation, the coexistence. It is in the coexistence that the nurse's biography, including her being a role, has a sense and meaning that we need to understand.

The Nursing Project

Schutz (1970) describes man's involvement in life in terms of acting in the outer world, and specifies that we are most fully interested in life, "wide-awake," in activity that reaches toward and modifies the world.

Nursing is a project, an attention to life. The nursing project and the nurse's role is one way to exist in the world. In wide-awakeness, the attention and involvement is vibrant; but, in any case, the nurse finds it possible to integrate time, realize the totality of herself, communicate with others, and organize space around her through her nursing. Or at least this becomes possible for her in work. Rather than depleting her energies, an aware involvement in nursing work gives them form and expression.

The knowledge the nurse brings to her work, the meanings she brings to and finds in the nursing situation, constitute the social situation she is involved in as much as they show her the way to involvement. The nurse has choices in the perspective she assumes in the world. In this way, the nurse has power over the nursing reality that is constituted by her. The nurse chooses and is chosen by the world.

This has particular relevance in nursing education. Nurse educators transmit a nursing culture to students. We teach them what nursing is, who nurses are, and the character of nursing situations. In short, we teach them a nursing perspective. When viewed as an introduction to a project that will determine students' perceptions, this process of socialization points to a number of educational concerns. Precisely what is a nursing perspective? And how is this perspective transmitted? Does the traditionally early focus on nursing's procedural skills in curricula effectively introduce students to the nursing perspective? Perhaps the nursing perspective is transmitted most effectively in nursing service after the student graduates. Perhaps our teaching methods interfere with, more than guide, the student toward the world in a nursing project. We may need to try new approaches to facilitate students' taking on that perspective which allows nursing to exist for them.

In view of the potential and need for diversity within the nursing perspective, what attention is given to the individual student's biography and its blend with the nursing perspective? What alternatives are extended to students to create a personal style that reflects a unique integration of their lives? It seems particularly relevant to examine socialization with reference to the presence of choices when considering students' developmental requirements. They are learning not only to be nurses, but also to exist in other projects. The youth of our students may argue for postponement of learning ambitions expressed in curricular objectives at this level.

There may be generational differences in the nursing perspective. The particular organization a nurse brings to her experience in terms of time is influenced by her idea of nursing's past, present, and future. A young nurse, for example, is largely limited to others' presentations of what nursing has been. The attention a nursing curriculum gives to nursing history can, in this sense, have an influence on the young nurse's integration of the past dimension of time in her work. To the degree that the nurse is isolated from nursing's past, she will be less able to be "wide-awake," invested in her project of nursing.

The same might be said for the present and future dimensions of time. Wide-awakeness requires a thorough communication with other nurses in their presents and ideas of their futures. Continuous exposure to other nurses' experiences and individual prespectives becomes a priority when viewed as requisite to individual nurse integration in her nursing work. In order to facilitate students' participation in meaningful dialogue, educators need to help them learn to listen effectively—to enter into discussion that frees them momentarily from themselves.

Personal integration and self-actualization in a phenomenological view are the outcomes of being aware and involved in the world through one's projects. Rather than bringing one's self to the nursing situation, it is through the nursing situation that one's self exists. There is no conflict between role and self in living forward. Although there seem to be thematic constancies in the nurse role and nursing perspective, these can be known only through consideration of the many individuated projects. The individual nurse's self-realization is significant in this sense not only for herself, but also for the meaning it lends to other nurses as they locate themselves in the world.

Detailed descriptions of competencies that prescribe being contradict the nature of making one's relation to the world through the nursing project. Nurse educators might open curricula in new directions to allow students to find their own integrations, enlightened by knowing the existence of other nurses.

However, the nurse educator's reality is not the student's. Although we may find new and more effective ways of presenting our realities to one another, this will not make the relation for anyone else. It can shape and clarify the nature of the nursing project. It can stimulate students' attention to nursing and accompany them in the form of meanings they assign to their nursing experiences. It can become an episode in the student's personal history. Yet if students are to realize themselves, the manner in which these meanings are arranged and ordered in their lives must not be predefined.

In experience, nurses are presented in perception with a simultaneity, a totality, in which neither the nurse nor the patient appear as objects. The other is accessible by a mutual living forward in simultaneous activity. Merleau-Ponty (1962) explains that "perception of others is anterior to, and the condition of" (p. 352), observations of others. Coexistence with patients is the foundation of the observations nurses make about them. Knowing the patient as an existence is experienced in the relation one has to the world; and is accessible through the ways the patient appears to us in perception. In order to appreciate the patient as a person, we need to focus on the patient's appearance in our perception. Further, the attempt to recover original perception in nursing facilitates a human encounter in which the nurse is revealed as a person.

The nurse's role with its knowledge, skills, and perspective is, according to Merleau-Ponty (1962), a "voluntary adoption of a position" (p. 355), from which truths are constructed. Informed by her experience in coexistence, the nurse can assume her role, constructing objective understandings which are continuous with lived reality. This is accomplished by disciplined reflection and active efforts to increase awareness, assume new perspectives, and perceive anew.

Modes of Awareness in Nursing

How do nurses become aware of their experiences? It has been noted that science gives us a mode of awareness by taking up a position in the world that objectifies the world. This is possible because we can turn back on experience in a reflective mode and think about it. Turning back on experience with concepts, constructs, models, and theories, we assume a position in relation to experience. This perspective in a scientific approach focuses experience in a particular way, according to the lens of the theoretical framework in use. The scientific theory sediments experience, and the observations it produces are an interpreted reality.

In nursing practice, as well as in nursing research, our observations of the nursing situation are sedimented in this way. This enables the nurse to bring scientific knowledge and techniques to the nursing situation, and to use these in the interest of the patient's recovery or well-being. To the extent that the nurse relies exclusively on the scientific mode of awareness, she treats the patient and herself as objects. In the absence of other modes of awareness, the nurse dehumanizes the patient and herself.

Nurses reach toward the world through their roles. Acting in the world, they are in simultaneous contact with the world and self in nursing experience. What modes of awareness are possible for nurses by virtue of being present in a situation shared with patients? Scientific, intuitive, empathic, imaginative, and reflective modes of awareness will be discussed briefly to indicate their value for nurses and students of nursing.

First, there is scientific awareness. The phenomena toward which consciousness is directed in nursing are the patient and his or her circumstances. In communication with the patient, the nurse intends toward the simultaneity of a reciprocal activity. She coexists now in the "we" of nurse and patient. The nurse-patient relationship, then, is another phenomenon which appears in the nurse's perception.

In turning back on her experience to reveal her perception, the nurse may adopt the mode of *knowing about* the patient and his or her circumstance. The nurse recalls facts about anxiety, for example, recognizing the patient's behavior as evidence of anxiety. Based on her observations of the patient and her theoretical knowledge about behavior, she analyzes the facts available to her. Turning back to her experience with these facts, the nurse constructs objective knowledge based on an interpreted reality.

If the nurse takes up a position in the world that directs her attention to self as object, she may also make observations about herself. The nurse may, for example, observe that she felt a pounding sensation in her chest or a lumpy sensation in her throat, and recognize this as evidence of anxiety. In the context of the patient's anxious behavior, the nurse may observe that her anxiety is a reaction to the patient. From there, the nurse will concern herself with identifying the cause or source of the anxiety, and with judging the appropriate response.

Some nurses attest to an intuitive sense in clinical practice. Intuition is, like other modes, a perspectival sense of meaning. In phenomenology, intuiting is an insight attained, in Merleau-Ponty's (1964) phrase, by "bringing out of my experience all that it implies, in thematizing what I have lived through at this time" (p. 54). It is the natural attitude of the nurse at those times when she is most open to her experiences, prior to categorizing and analyzing it.

Empathizing is a particularly interesting mode of awareness in nursing. An insight into the patient's experiences as if they were one's own, this mode is not dependent on the patient's description of his or her experience. Rather, nursing's participation with patients in daily living experiences presents nurses with multiple occasions to know their patients in this way. Considered from the perspective of coexistence in the nurse-patient relationship, empathic moments come close to revealing perception itself.

Imagining is an allied mode of awareness of potential value to nurses in their work. As Merleau-Ponty (1964) has stated:

> To imagine is always to make something absent appear in the present, to give a magical quasipresence to an object that is not there. (p. 60)

There is in imagination a reaching toward the phenomenon and the setting up of a relation with it. This mode of awareness relies on lived experience to reveal analogues of the absent object. As a means of freeing oneself from the limits of a priori perspectives, imagining holds promise for nurses in view of the emphasis on understanding others.

According to Schutz (1970, pp. 168–178), the aim of understanding another person has two meanings: understanding one's lived experience of the other and understanding another's lived experience. Genuine understanding is concerned not merely with the display of grief or anger in the patient's conduct, for example, but with the patient's experience of suffering or anger. Imagining the experience of suffering or anger enables us to transcend perception of the patient as object by calling on our own experiences of suffering and anger. We are able to do this because we have experienced the patient in coexistence: the patient is one whose relation to the world is constituted like our own. And it is through imagination that we are able to make our own similar experience appear in perception.

Our past experience of suffering may have been in fantasy, as in reading a novel, but even a vicarious experience of suffering is helpful in understanding another's actual experience of suffering. The implications of this for nursing are obvious. First, the nurses's experiences in the world are seen to be a fundamental resource. Second, there is enormous value for nurses in literature and the arts as a means of expanding their experiences vicariously. However, to focus exclusively on the patient's behavior as a manifestation of his or her human experience is clearly an inadequate basis upon which to found an *understanding* of him or her.

According to Spiegelberg (1975), "imaginative self-transposal" (pp. 46–53) is a means of increasing our ability to see through another's eyes. It is a kind of disciplined imagination, subject to clues and rules, similar to that used in science and art. By combining personal observations of the patient and biographical facts about the patient, the nurse can imaginatively assume the patient's perspective in the world. Carefully observing the patient's situation and the patient's behavior in that situation both contain clues which the nurse uses to test her imaginative experience by. There is, then, according to Spiegelberg, a requirement to "shuttle back and forth between our own understanding self and that of the other."

The patient's descriptions of his or her perspective are yet another source of clues that must be used in a continuous revision or reconstruction of this vicarious experience. In this regard, the patient's ability to describe his or her experience will influence the quantity and quality of these clues. The traditional interview may be an insufficient technique for nurses in data collection of this type.

Role-playing, which is often used in nursing education, is another technique by which nursing students can make a relation to their patients. By having students experience blindness or sit in a wheelchair or wear a cast, educators have guided students towards an understanding of patients' experiences. From the phenomenological view, this is intending toward the world in a particular way, taking up a particular perspective in the world, so as to discover this way of existing. According to Spiegelberg (1975), this approach to sharing in "parallel experience" (p. 47) is one way to expand our grasp of phenomena not given in direct experience, although its artificial and escapable quality does limit its value.

In the reflective mode of awareness, the last to be considered here, meaning is determined by the perspective given in a relation to the world (Merleau-Ponty, 1964, pp. 64–68). For the nurse, the reflective mode has a singular aim: to disengage as much as possible from her "historicity" in order to reveal her perception more fully. One can "stand over against" his or her existence in experience by recalling experience and thinking back on it. Wondering why one feels nostalgic when remembering his or her home town, or why he or she likes a painting, are examples of this kind of reflection. In the strict sense given to this by phenomenology, the elements of autobiographical reflection are methodically and rigorously disengaged from one's concern and attention. According to Zaner (1970), the purpose of this radical reflection is to allow the inquirer to view his or her engagement by stepping back from it.

I do not propose here that nurses can practically perform such a radical disengagement from the components of their roles and the requirements of the nursing project. Rather, I suggest that it is useful at times to peel away some of our suppositions about the world, and look again at our experiences. The reflective mode can be used relatively, with the intention of recognizing and appreciating the nurse, the patient, and the patient's circumstance as a complex human reality that is not split in experience.

There are multiple modes of awareness available to nurses that will serve to increase our understanding of nursing reality. None of these, including scientific awareness, is sufficient in itself to inform nursing practice. In the phenomenological perspective, a fundamental premise is that the nurse can enrich her gaze and become more wide-awake by using all the modes given in her humanness. Since we are situated and biographically determined in the world, numerous means of expanding awareness of our immediate reality will only serve to enhance the nursing project. We can become more aware of ourselves and what we live through with patients. We can consciously clarify the concepts we use to orient the world around us, and select and create those that are consistent with nursing reality.

Means of Expanding Awareness in Nursing Education

The concern in nursing with delivering care to others focuses our attention on describing and understanding nursing from two points of view: the nurse's experience of the nurse-patient relationship and the patient's experience in his or her circumstance.

We need to ask of the nursing perspective what it gives to experience and what it takes from it. Finding meaningful ways for nurses to present their experiences to one another is prerequisite toward this end. Meaning, of course, is generated in nursing experience. Our concepts about nursing need, then, to take direction from the experience of nursing. In modes of awareness that reduce the layers of meaning superimposed on experience by our values, beliefs, and knowledge, we can expect to find experience presented in ways that adhere more closely to lived experience. Intuiting, empathizing, imagining, and reflecting awarenesses each seizes the world from a particular point of view and in a particular grasp of *meaning in experience*.

When we approach a nursing situation with an assessment format, with the intention to observe a patient, we treat him as an object in a split reality. We collect facts about this object-patient, and he or she is displayed in awareness as an object rather than as another existence. Focusing the coexistence of nurse and patient aims at understanding and responding humanly to patients' experiences. As interpretive agents of experience, nurses need phenomenological approaches to their experiences as lived: to clarify the perspectives we adopt and the meanings they bring to the nursing situation.

The nurse's log of her experience is recognized and used as an aid to the nurse's becoming more aware of her practice. The log is, however, often confined to students' experience in psychiatric nursing. From the phenomenological point of view, the value in the log resides in the occasion it provides for the nurse to render her experience and to enter into dialogue with her own expression. This unique feature of the log commends it to continued and expanded use in nursing. There is a new structuring of experience that occurs when recalling and using language to describe it that the audio- or video-recorder does not accomplish on its own.

The case study design in nursing research is also limited to an essentially academic mode where it is frequently used as a model for clinical nursing course requirements. Particularly in conjunction with experimental and survey research designs, the case study warrants reconsideration of its potential uses. As in the log, the case study has immediate value to the nurse who expresses her experience in this way as well as to those who act in dialogue with it. In the case study, there is an additional opportunity to blend modes of awareness. In some case studies, nurses have moved among several perspectives in reflection, commenting first with one layer of meaning and then with another. Found occasionally in students' unpublished work, such variety of expression in the case study reveals an unexplored way to knowing about nursing.

Nurses' anecdotal reports of their experiences are another form of valuable expression usually overlooked. These reports bear a similarity to the log and case study, but are distinct from them in a typical style of spontaneous storytelling. Frequently, the nurse's prompting to tell her story seems to be generated by the experience itself. The stories are of achievement and success in the nurse-patient relationship, and are rendered in the nurse's natural attitude in the world. There are typically no theoretical formulations or footnotes to document her expression. The nurse simply and clearly tells us how her experience looks to her.

From a scientific point of view, the anecdotal report is an undisciplined remembrance of the nurse-patient relationship. From the phenomenological view, it is of value to us as a reflection on and rendering of that remembrance. The anecdotal report is, like all expressions of lived reality, a reconstruction of reality. It gives experience new meaning and enters it in the cultural world of nursing. It can be explored in this sense of revealing nursing perspectives, and in recognition that our understanding will always be incomplete. There is in the log, case study, and anecdotal report, then, a tacit license for the nurse to vary from the scientific perspective in a search for meaning. This license might be extended to nurses explicitly in a solicitation of their descriptions of experience.

Searching for ways to call on new awarenesses for nurses, we might, for example, ask nurses to respond to art or poetry or novels, to reflect on the similarities and contrasts in others' realities and their own. In all of this, we can expect to reveal nursing perspectives, to signify meanings thematically, and to construct profiles of nursing reality that take their sense from a disciplined reflection on nurses' commitment to the world in the nursing project.

Like reactions to art, nurses' expressions in the art modes are indirect communications which have the special value of provoking new awareness within a disruption of familiar meanings. We are drawn to look at the world from a new position in it, and to constitute new

Table 3
Nursing Education Phenomena

The nurse-patient relationship.
Patient and his circumstance as object.
Nurse (self) as object.
Nurse's experiences in the world.
Vicarious experience.
Patient's description of his experience.
Nurse and patient indirect expressions.

Table 4
Means of Expanding Awareness in Nursing

Expanded data base formats.
Clarified nursing perspectives.
Nursing prose: logs, case studies, and anecdotes.
Dialogue.
Fictional and autobiographical accounts of experience.
Response to art.
Artistic expression.

meanings. The incompleteness of truth is bridged somewhat in this way, as we add new profiles to reality.

To summarize this review of the implications of phenomenological philosophy for nursing, Table 3 lists nursing phenomena to focus in our curricula and Table 4 provides an indication of experiences and materials that would be relevant to such an aim.

CONCLUSION

For many of us in nursing education, the humanistic tradition is an irresistible current in a time replete with evidence of a need for renewal of humanistic loyalties. Toward this end, the following recommendations are offered.

1. Identify the nurse-patient relationship as a central curricular theme.
2. Use a wider variety of modes of awareness to interpret realities of lived experience.

3. Define the nursing database to include nurse *and* patient perception.
4. Expand the use of the humanities in the nursing process.
5. Develop nursing as an individual project.
6. Develop dialogue as a means of carrying individuals' nursing projects forward.
7. Expand the use of qualitative data in research and evaluation projects.
8. Blend the nurse/researcher roles.
9. Balance faculty composition to include multiple perspectives.
10. Scrutinize conflicts between the aims and means of professional and liberal education.

REFERENCES

Benner, P. (1983). Uncovering the knowledge embedded in clinical practice. *Image, 15*, 36–41.

Merleau-Ponty, M. (1964). *The primacy of perception* (J. Edie, Trans.). Evanston: Northwestern University Press.

Merleau-Ponty, M. (1962). *Phenomenology of perception* (C. Colin, Trans.). New York: Humanities Press.

Munhall, P., & Oiler, C. (1986). *Nursing research: A qualitative perspective*. Norwalk, CT: Appleton-Century-Crofts.

Oiler, C. (1986). Qualitative methods: Phenomenology. In P. Moccia, *New Approaches to Theory Development*. New York: National League for Nursing.

Oiler, C. (1982) The Phenomenological approach in nursing research. *Nursing Research, 31*, 79–81.

Omery, A. (1983). Phenomenology: A method for nursing research. *Advances in Nursing Science, 5*, 49–63.

Orlando, I. (1961). *The dynamic nurse-patient relationship*. New York: G.P. Putnam's Sons.

Parse, R. (1981). *Man-living-health: A theory of nursing*. New York: John Wiley and Sons.

Paterson, J., & Zderad, L. (1976). *Humanistic nursing*. New York: John Wiley and Sons.

Ray, M. (1985). A philosophical method to study nursing phenomena. In M. Leininger, *Qualitative research methods in nursing*. New York: Grune & Stratton.

Schutz, A. (1970). *On phenomenology and social relations*. Chicago: University of Chicago Press.

Spiegelberg, H. (1975). *Doing phenomenology*. The Hague, Netherlands: Martinus-Nijhoff.

Ujhely, G. (1968). *Determinants of the nurse-patient relationship*. New York: Springer Publishing.

Watson, J. (1985). Human science and human care: A theory of nursing. Norwalk, CT: Appleton-Century-Crofts.

Wiedenbach, E. (1965). *Clinical nursing: A helping art*. New York: Springer Publishing.

Zaner, R. (1970). *The way of phenomenology*. Indianapolis, IN: Pegasus.

BIBLIOGRAPHY

Cohen, M. (1987). A historical overview of the phenomenological movement. *Image, 19*, 31–34.

Denton, D. (Ed.). (1974). *Existentialism and phenomenology in education*. New York: Teachers College Press.

Dewey, J. (1958). *Art as experience*. New York: G. P. Putnam's Sons.

Dossey, L. (1982). *Space, time and medicine*. Boulder, CO: Shabhala Publications, Inc.

Greene, M. (1978). *Landscapes of learning*. New York: Teachers College Press.

Greene, M. (1973). *Teacher as stranger*. Belmont, CA: Wadsworth Publishing Co., Inc.

Nisbet, R. (1976). *Sociology as an art form*. New York: Oxford University Press.

Oiler, C. (1980). *A phenomenological perspective in nursing*. Unpublished doctoral dissertation, Teachers College, Columbia University, New York.

Oiler, C. (1983). Nursing reality as reflected in nurses' poetry. *Perspectives in Psychiatric Care, 21*, 81–89.

Reeder, F. (1987). The phenomenological movement. *Image, 19*, 150–152.

Spiegelberg, H. (1976). *The phenomenological movement, vols. I and II*. The Hague, Netherlands: Martinus Nijhoff.

Strasser, S. (1963). *Phenomenology and the human sciences*. Pittsburgh: Duquesne University Press.

Zderad, L., & Belcher, H. (1968). *Developing behavioral concepts in nursing*. Atlanta, GA: Southern Regional Education Board.

6

Innovations in Clinical Teaching

Alma S. Woolley and Susan E. Costello

The rapid transformation of the health care delivery system has been described from a variety of perspectives: those of organized medicine and nursing; those of consumer and payor groups; and those of policy-makers at the local, state, and federal levels. Until recently, nursing education has responded only incrementally to these system changes. Joel (1987) cites a recent survey conducted by MARNA in which only 52 percent of the nurse educators who participated indicated that curricula had been modified in response to the changing health care environment. Indeed, 55 percent stated that they saw no need to change.

In this paper, we will explore some clinical teaching strategies that are responsive to the radical alterations now taking place in the health care delivery system. These alterations include

- changes in reimbursement strategies, such as prospective payment and diagnosis related groupings (DRGs);
- an increase in the market share of managed care plans, such as preferred provider organizations (PPOs) and health management organizations (HMOs);
- increased demand from consumers and payors for high-quality cost-effective care; and
- Increased attention to health promotion.

These changes have had numerous important consequences, including

- greater use of community-based providers, such as free-standing radiology and diagnostic centers, clinics, and office-based providers;
- development of same-day services, both free-standing and hospital-based, for minor surgery and diagnostic procedures;
- use of "day of services," which means that patients are admitted on the day a procedure is to be done and that they first arrive on the patient care unit *after* the procedure has been completed;
- expansion of the home care industry, including providers of home nursing care, manufacturers of medical equipment, and pharmaceutical vendors;
- increased acuity of patients in acute care facilities; and
- Decreased length of patient stay, which results in a greater need for effective use of inpatient time, early discharge planning, and patient and family education.

The profession as a whole must respond to these changes and their effects, and nursing education in particular must respond as well. The demand for more and better prepared nurses is heard daily. The urgent questions, however, remain: how do we more adequately prepare nurses, and what would a responsive curriculum look like? Specifically, what innovations in clinical teaching would best enable graduates to practice effectively in today's health care market?

PURPOSES OF CLINICAL TEACHING

Clinical teaching has several purposes. It enables the learner to integrate the knowledge and skills associated with caring for patients. In addition, it gives students the opportunity to internalize the role of the nurse as caregiver.

Benner (1984) has adapted the Dreyfus model of skill acquisition to describe the process by which clinical nursing skill is developed. In this model, an individual passes through five levels of proficiency in the acquisition and development of skills: (1) novice, (2) advanced beginner, (3) competent, (4) proficient, and (5) expert. The levels are distinguished first by a move from "reliance on abstract principles to the use of past concrete experience as paradigms" and second by a shift from a view of a clinical situation as a mass of discrete bits of data to a view of the situation as a single multifaceted context, within which the more relevant parts can be emphasized. According to Benner, clinical experience enables the student to move from being a novice who relies on abstract principles learned in class to being an advanced beginner, a new graduate, who uses past experiences with patient situations as paradigms. During the clinical part of the nursing curriculum, the student gains the experience necessary for integrating details of care and clinical observations into a larger, more sophisticated view of patient situations.

The main objective of clinical experience, therefore, is to ensure that students (novices) acquire the ability to provide nursing care to patients at the advanced beginner level; many more years are needed to reach competent, proficient, and expert status. The current changes in the health care delivery system challenge us to evaluate our current methodology and explore new means of achieving this objective.

Developing a Focus on Process

Joel (1987) has recommended that in order to avoid being a "content-laden curriculum" (p. 20), nursing education should be process-focused rather than content-focused. This idea is not a new one, but it may take on a different meaning in today's rapidly changing health care environment.

Until recently, we could expect to introduce students to most if not all of the major content of nursing through courses in medical, surgical, pediatric, obstetric, psychiatric, and community health nursing, which were designed to prepare them to provide care to patients with problems in these areas. Integrated curricular models have attempted to modify the theoretical portion of the curriculum in such a way as to focus on common problems or concepts of nursing. In the clinical laboratory, however, we still try to match students' assignments to the concepts concurrently being discussed in the didactic portion of the course.

We have long known how difficult it is to match didactic and clinical assignments, but we have not really asked ourselves whether this should be the focus of our energies. If our goal is to ensure that the student assimilates the process of caring for patients by integrating the necessary knowledge and skills, then a greater portion of clinical time should be spent teaching the student to apply the nursing process in clinical situations. This means teaching the *process of caring* for pediatric or surgical patients, rather than the specific nursing interventions for pediatric patients with this or that medical diagnosis. It is by working closely with more skilled practitioners, observing the use of the process, and building a bank of situational experience on which to base future clinical judgments that the student learns this process.

ATTAINMENT OF CLINICAL OBJECTIVES

As advanced beginners, the graduates of a basic nursing program are expected to be able to assess the health and nursing needs of clients and formulate nursing diagnoses on the basis of this assessment. They should also be able to develop and implement a plan of care that builds on the patient's strengths to resolve the identified nursing needs. Finally, they should be able to establish criteria for evaluating the effects of the interventions and determining whether revision of the plan is necessary.

Traditional Methods

Assessment. Traditionally, we have evaluated students' capacity for accurate assessment by providing them with patient assignments before the assigned clinical experience and requiring them to identify the patients' most likely deviations from norms, strengths and limitations, and nursing needs. On their arrival in the clinical area, students thoroughly assess the patients and either validate or revise the plan of care. This procedure assumes that students will be able to predict patients' nursing needs on the basis of medical diagnoses and limited demographic data and that they will have sufficient access to patients to do assessments during the first few hours of the clinical day.

Until recently the average length of hospitalization was seven to ten days; thus, it was reasonable to assume that students would have the opportunity for several contacts with their assigned patients. Now that the average length of stay is between five and seven days, this assumption can no longer be made. Decreased length of stay has led to tighter scheduling of inpatient time, which means that availability of patients to students is less predictable. With the traditional Tuesday/Thursday clinical schedule, students are often assigned to different patients each day. Consequently, they do not always have the opportunity to identify and fill in gaps in the nursing assessment.

What is more, it can no longer be assumed that clients' needs are likely to be predictable. Patients in acute care settings rarely have a single primary diagnosis: multiple comorbidities are the norm rather than the exception.

Planning and Implementation. It is with respect to planning and implementation skills that the need to change our clinical teaching strategies is most obvious. Traditionally, we have taught these skills by requiring students, as part of their preclinical preparation, to write hypothetical nursing care plans for their assigned patients based on information provided by clinical faculty members and on the conceptual framework of the program. In the clinical setting, we expect students to evaluate the appropriateness of these plans, revise them accordingly, and initiate the appropriate interventions.

Here too, the increasing unpredictability of patient needs and the decreasing length of stay pose significant problems. Furthermore, it is probable that care plans for the patients already exist, and it is probable that the school of nursing's conceptual model may not agree with that of the clinical agency. Many agencies have elected to use manual or automated standardized plans of care or nursing protocols rather than create wholly unique care plans for each patient. Given the decreasing length of stay, it is essential that plans of care be established at admission, followed closely thereafter, and revised as often as necessary. These plans must not only meet immediate acute care needs but also prepare patients and families to provide care at home. With the advent of case management ("second-generation primary nursing") the idea that students ought to spend their time developing independent plans of care becomes increasingly problematic. Many case management programs are moving away from the traditional nursing care plan and relying increasingly on nursing protocols and nursing orders. All nursing care providers are expected to follow the nursing orders and negotiate any changes with the case manager.

Because of the limited clinical exposure available to students, nursing curricula have made heavy use of the care plan as a teaching tool. Care planning allows students to explore all the interventions that might be appropriate for a particular patient. Unfortunately, this exploration usually leads to the identification of more interventions than can or should be carried out. The ultimate outcome of student care planning may be nothing more than cognitive dissonance.

An additional concern arising from our current approach is that since students are expected to focus on the total care of only one and sometimes two patients, the opportunities for them to acquire the broad situational experience they need to make clinical judgments are severely limited.

Evaluation. Traditionally, we have assumed that students would have repeated contact with their assigned patients and thus would have ample opportunity both to implement and to evaluate the effectiveness of their interventions. This is certainly no longer the case. Students are currently required to include in their proposed care plans the specific criteria they will use to evaluate the effectiveness of the plan. It is thought that in the clinical setting they may also be able to evaluate the effects of their own interventions and participate in evaluating the effectiveness of the staff's plan of care. Unfortunately, for the reasons noted earlier, students have increasingly less opportunity to evaluate the long-term or even the intermediate effects of their interventions.

In light of the enormous systemic and environmental changes taking place in health care delivery, we must question whether these traditional approaches to integrating knowledge and skills are still viable and ask ourselves if there might be better ways of reaching our clinical education goals.

ALTERNATIVE APPROACHES TO ATTAINING OBJECTIVES

Alternative Clinical Settings

Many of the changes in acute care necessitate increased collaboration between outpatient and inpatient providers. Preadmission testing is performed in outpatient settings, such as office practices and diagnostic centers. The results are communicated to the inpatient providers, who are then free to determine what interventions are required. Thus, placing students in outpatient settings might help them to improve their skills in assessment and diagnosis.

There are numerous other clinical settings, such as managed care programs, HMOs, and group practices, that are worthy of exploration. These alternatives to independent primary care settings offer nursing students an excellent opportunity to develop their assessment and diagnostic skills. These providers have a considerable investment in health promotion and illness prevention as well as a strong interest in early diagnosis and treatment. Working with them would allow students to see other patients besides those with acute multisystem health problems; it would give them the chance to provide care to clients across the health–illness spectrum and participate in the management of a greater variety of health problems than they could in acute care settings. To date, access to these providers—who also, by the way, offer excellent opportunities for faculty practice—has not been adequately explored by schools of nursing. Students and faculty members together could actively engage in the management of members' care.

The chance to hone the skills of assessment and diagnosis is also available in public clinics for the indigent, shelters for the homeless, and rescue missions (Woolley, 1985). Physical and psychosocial assessment skills can be practiced in these settings, in which a wide range of health deviations is readily found. As the number of un- or underinsured people steadily rises, local and regional governments and charitable organizations are setting up more clinics to meet the growing needs of this group. Participation in these efforts is an excellent way for schools of nursing to meet their community service obligations: students can work towards their clinical objective while contributing to their communities.

Computer Simulation

Much of the computer software currently on the market provides alternative approaches to the teaching of some components of clinical nursing. Several authoring programs are available that allow instructors to design course- and content-specific care planning simulations that guide students through the development of care plans for patients with various needs. It is possible to program the option of evaluating the expected outcome of each intervention into these simulations, which allows students to revise their original plans.

There are already many programs that have organized essential content into self-paced modules that contain corresponding college and clinical laboratory objectives. Using such programs would free a great deal of teaching time for discussion and clarification, which might eliminate the mass lectures, frantic note-taking, and game-playing about what will and will not be on exams that now seem inseparable from nursing education. This would encourage greater emphasis on developing competence in the nursing process and in clinical judgment, that is, on locating and using information rather than on storing it.

Laboratory Simulation

Infante (1975) has been advocating the use of laboratory simulation for many years. Crucial to her argument is the idea that there is a clear difference between "caring for clients" and "learning how to care for clients." She suggests that students can effectively learn how to care for clients—i.e., the psychomotor skills of caring—in the college laboratory. They can then proceed to the clinical setting, especially in the early part of the program, to observe, test hypotheses, and assist in specific parts of care. They are assigned to learning activities, not to patients. For example, a student who has learned to do ostomy care in the college laboratory could go to the clinical laboratory to observe nurses actually providing such care to patients of varying age, weight, body structure, and self-care ability. The student could then compare the different techniques used, ask questions, and assist the practitioner with the procedure.

Infante's work, though influential, has not had the impact it might have. Imagine how much better prepared students would be if they could use a combination of computer-assisted clinical simulations, interactive video, and a college laboratory to learn how to care before they actually care for clients.

Expanded Clinical Teaching

Nursing students need better access to patients, and we need better collaboration between nursing service and nursing education. Education and service must work together to expand the clinical opportunities available to students, perhaps starting with flexible hours, days, and assignments. Once students have learned how to plan care for patients and how to provide this care, all under the guidance of faculty members, the next thing they need to learn in the clinical setting is the actual process of caring for patients. They also need to assimilate sufficient situational experience to acquire an adequate database for making clinical judgments, thereby moving from novice to advanced beginner status.

Use of agency personnel as clinical teaching assistants or preceptors for undergraduate nursing students is not a new practice, but it has usually been limited to the senior year in a clinical elective course. Some schools of nursing, such as that at the University of Colorado, have been exploring the extension of this practice to other levels of the curriculum (Phillips & Kaempfer, 1987). In most cases, the clinical teaching assistants assume responsibility for direct clinical teaching of students under the supervision of a member of the school of nursing faculty. Typically, they provide clinical instruction to a small group of students one or two days a week. Although this results in increased collaboration between education and service, each student still provides care to only one patient during each clinical exposure.

Perhaps it is time to consider expanding these collaborative models and to experiment with placing each student with a carefully selected (according to stated criteria), highly motivated staff nurse/teaching assistant on a one-to-one basis. The student would help care for the nurse's four to six assigned patients, the staff nurse would help the student to achieve the objectives specified by the faculty; and a faculty member would provide teaching supervision to the nurse.

The student's overall clinical objective would be to learn the process of caring for adults and children with health care deficits. Such learning could be fostered in several ways. For example, students enrolled in a course in the developing family could be assigned to work with a pediatric nurse for part of the semester and with an obstetric nurse for the other part; students in a complex nursing problems course could be assigned to nurses working in critical care areas. These approaches would give students greater exposure to a variety of clinical situations and help them to develop a broad base for clinical judgments. Because of increased exposure to technology, the students would also be more likely to develop their technical competence. The emphasis would not be on how to care, which would be attended to in the college laboratory, but rather on the "caring for" process in the actual clinical setting.

Students could also be granted more scheduling flexibility. If they do not always have to go to the clinical laboratory at specific times, they will have a wider choice of times in which to take their non-nursing classes. The common scenario in which all nursing majors take English or philosophy together merely because they are the only classes that fit into their rigid schedule is clearly undesirable.

Moreover, the traditional senior practicum experience could be spent working with a "case manager" to plan the course of patients' admissions. In schools where case management is not in use, students could be assigned to work with a patient who will need home care; they could plan and evaluate the continuum of care and perhaps even make home visits. In either case, students would be expected to look beyond the immediate admission and focus their attention on the client's long-term health care needs.

Pre- and Post-Conferences

If clinical hours and assignments are made more flexible, the concept of pre- and post-conferences will have to be modified. This concept was introduced by Matheney (1969) as a key part of her plan for producing technical nurses in two years. Matheney believed that if the objectives for the day were made clear to a group of students, each student could then achieve the objectives with a different patient, and that if what was achieved was shared at the end of the day, each student would have a broader learning experience. Many baccalaureate programs use pre- and post-conferences for similar purposes (Wolf & O'Driscoll, 1979); the group post-conference is probably more commonly employed than the pre-conference.

There is, however, no real evidence that this particular methodology is effective. Matheney certainly envisioned these conferences as more than weary show-and-tell wrap-ups. She expected each instructor to be planning the conference while simultaneously overseeing and demonstrating the care of 8 or 10 or 12 patients to as many novices. Unfortunately, the onset of hunger pangs often combines with the effects of a 5 AM wakeup call to make post-conferences less than ideal for students and teachers alike. It would not be difficult to plan a better time for group discussion, sharing, and problem solving. Weekly clinical rounds for all involved—faculty, clinical teaching assistants, and students—might better serve the purpose of broadening students' learning.

Case Management

If the graduates of our program are to be case managers as well as direct caregivers, we will have to give students the opportunity to explore this role. They will need to know that, as professional care managers, they must be able to delegate tasks, supervise, and evaluate less skilled workers.

At Georgetown University a group of senior nursing students is spending a community health semester in a public clinic where a large number of patients have tested positive for the human immune virus (HIV). The students do baseline assessments, provide health teaching and support to patients returning for follow-up, and make home visits to oversee and evaluate care being provided by "personal care aides" and "chore aides." In their last semester, a group of students who have chosen this setting for their senior elective will design an evaluation system that the agency will use to monitor care and predict resource needs. They will also work in greater depth with terminally ill AIDS patients, lend support to families and caregivers, and gain experience in the management of scarce resources. Several faculty members also practice in this setting and conduct a support group for families.

ACCREDITATION CONCERNS

Whenever we discuss modifications in the content or methodology of our curricula, we must try to ensure that the changes we are considering will not keep our programs from meeting the relevant accreditation criteria. Fortunately, these criteria can be met in many different ways, and they are revised frequently in response to changing educational practices. Examination of some of the terms that often appear in accreditation criteria and competency statements may help us to see the need for changes in clinical teaching.

Faculty-Related Terms

Faculty-Student Ratio. One of the critical variables in the NLN accreditation process is the faculty-student ratio. A small ratio is traditionally considered an indicator that the school has adequate resources. Theoretically, maintaining a ratio of one instructor to eight or ten students provides the close supervision of clinical learning that we have come to associate with nursing programs in institutions of higher education. It helps to ensure that clinical hours are learning hours and that each student's progress or lack thereof is closely monitored, recorded, evaluated, and, when necessary, promptly remedied. It reduces student demands on nursing staff time and leaves the staff free to provide direct patient care. It protects students from exploitation by agencies concerned with meeting their own needs rather than those of the learner. On the other hand, it is this low ratio more than anything else that is responsible for the high cost of nursing education. It is this ratio that makes schools of nursing so labor-intensive, causes budgets to soar, and discourages parent institutions from providing support in tight fiscal situations.

Meanwhile, both students and agencies complain that students are usually able to care for only one patient per laboratory experience. The major reason for this, especially with patients who have complex problems, is that one instructor, however expert, really cannot cope with more than eight to ten novices *and* eight to ten sick patients. Realistically, even with an 8:1 ratio, there is not very much teaching time available for each student. If we start with six clinical hours and subtract pre- and post-conferences, lunch, and coffee breaks (for the students, that is), about four hours are left. Dividing this figure by eight students yields about a half hour per student and patient, per frantic instructor. Considering that part of that half hour is taken up in saying good morning to the patients, finding the students, and editing students' charts, little one-to-one teaching time is left. Consequently, instructors actually observe only a very small sample of each student's learning day.

We must ask ourselves, are there other ways of ensuring that students' experiences are primarily learning experiences, helping them to progress as far as they can, and making their transition to the reality of practice easier than it is now?

Professional Modeling. Another reason for a low faculty-student ratio is that it enables faculty members to provide demonstration and modeling of professional practice. Faculty members are the "supernurses" who know the patients, the staff, and the nursing procedures well enough to demonstrate them to students.

In earlier, and simpler times, this may have been quite possible. Indeed, there are still many nursing faculty members who, because of their own concomitant nursing practice, are able to accomplish this feat; however, there are just as many who are no longer able to do so. They are not in the agencies long enough or often enough to know the patients, the staff, and the intricate procedures and technologies in use. They do not usually attend inservice programs that offer updates on new procedures. The pressure to publish, to do research, to make presentations, to plan curricula, and to attend committee meetings crowd their week and prevent them from spending extra time in clinical activities. As good educators, however, they know what they do not know and are able to call on the staff for assistance when necessary. Consequently, the system survives.

We must ask ourselves, is there a way to reduce the labor-intensive costs of our programs while providing expert, knowledgeable practitioner role models for students at all times? Is there a better way of using faculty members prepared as specialists and educators, so that they are able to fulfill all facets of the academic role?

Role Change. Changes in nursing education will necessitate changes in faculty roles. If any of the alternative approaches I have described are implemented, some faculty members will find their role evolving into that of a master teacher. This role will extend beyond guiding nursing students to guiding all those involved in assisting students to acquire the knowledge and skills of advanced beginners. The faculty will plan and develop the students' laboratory activities, develop computer-assisted instruction (CAI) and clinical simulations, and make summative evaluative judgments about students' performance. They will plan learning activities to prepare staff nurse clinical teaching assistants and provide them with coaching and supervision. Closer association between staff and faculty will provide increased opportunities for joint clinical research projects.

Curriculum-Related Terms

Across the Life Cycle. Students are expected to care for clients in every stage of life, from birth to death, and to think of a client's particular place on that continuum as a conditioning factor in the person's nursing needs. Not long ago, it was not only possible but probable that students would be systematically assigned to clients in every age group, each with its particular set of maturational crises interacting with the health state.

Today, this is more difficult to do. Fewer children are admitted to acute care facilities, and fewer young and middle-aged adults are hospitalized. Although comparatively little gerontology course content is taught, most of the patients the students care for are elderly. In addition, more and more clients are developmentally disabled, which poses additional problems in assessing and planning care.

If we are to teach students about the health needs of persons all along the continuum, and not just at one end or the other, we must go where the clients are: schools, day care centers for the developmentally disabled, clinics, HMOs, and homes, where there are abundant opportunities for practicing assessment skills and teaching health care. At Georgetown University, some of the juniors have their psychiatric-mental health experience at a community facility for the dually diagnosed, that is, the developmentally disabled who also have a mental illness. A few years ago, we would not have sought out a facility like this.

Simple to Complex. Most curricula interpret this phrase to mean that students look first at one client, then at the family, and finally at the community. Is it realistic, though, even to talk about an individual without considering whether a family is present or not, or whether the client lives in suburbia, a nursing home, or a prison? Moreover, students find it difficult to move past the individual to an understanding of the context of illness and how it is influenced by environmental variables. With increased visiting hours, shorter stays, and the probability that continued care will be necessary after discharge, the family and community must be part of care from the very beginning, not just late-stage add-ons. It will be impossible for us to meet health needs in today's no longer simple society if we perpetuate this narrow stepwise approach in the curriculum.

Today, many programs are finding it increasingly difficult to meet the objectives of first-level courses, which include orientation to the hospital setting, practicing basic nursing procedures, and designing "simple" nursing systems for clients with "simple" nursing needs. The main reason this is so is that clients with "simple" problems are no longer languishing in hospital beds. The hospital population is now made up of more and more very sick people with complex needs.

Although new students cannot possibly care for such complex needs, they can help the nurses assigned to the patients with one or two tasks at a time—feeding, turning, positioning, explaining (*not* teaching, which is more complex) what will happen next, transferring, changing a dressing, and so on. In the course of the semester, the student could perform a series of simple nursing actions, while the graduate nurse retains responsibility for all the complex needs of the patient. The simple-to-complex approach can be used to guide mastery of specific tasks, but it is rarely applicable to assessing and planning care or to describing the complex wholeness we call health.

The simple-to-complex principle is also frequently given as the reason why students need to learn about health, in sometimes tedious detail, before studying illness. Some programs attempt to adhere to this principle by having students interact first with "healthy" clients. Besides finding this process less than exciting, novices are often unable to answer clients' questions or do any substantive health teaching, because they lack both classroom knowledge and situational experience.

Experience With Clients From Diverse Populations. "Clients from diverse populations" is usually interpreted to mean clients other than those in the natural habitat of the school. Unfortunately, there are still many programs that do not include a basic course in cultural anthropology that provides a framework for transcultural health care experiences. In the future, many of the clients who need nursing will have health practices, beliefs, and life styles very different from our own.

Many students in baccalaureate programs wish that they, like liberal arts majors, could spend part or all of their junior year abroad. Since this is not a real possibility for many or perhaps most nursing majors, could we not provide a transcultural semester at home, so that students could begin to develop an in-depth relationship with members of a different ethnic group? Obviously, this would be easier to do in an urban area, but there are actually very few areas in the United States where it would be impossible. Transcultural nursing has been around for more than 30 years, and we must take it seriously if we want to prepare our students for health care delivery in the 21st century.

EVALUATION

Evaluation of a Process-Focused Curriculum

Evaluation of clinical learning experiences has a "long and tortured history" (Woolley, 1977), and we will undoubtedly add several new chapters as we update our curricula for the health care delivery system of the future. In a process-as-content curriculum, what is evaluated is the student's ability to carry out the nursing process according to the terminal objectives of the program—i.e., diploma, associate degree, or baccalaureate.

Several extensive projects have been carried out within the last few years (Primm, 1986; Stull, 1986) that have delineated and differentiated the terminal competencies of graduates of associate degree and baccalaureate programs. These projects take the nursing process to be the basis of the care given by both types of graduates; they see the focus of each step as differing somewhat between the two types of practitioner but nonetheless complementary. These differentiated competency statements provide an overall guide for evaluation of students in both programs.

In a process-as-content curriculum, there are many ways of evaluating mastery of the process besides sampling behavior during direct care. We have only begun to make use of the simulation opportunities technology has made available. Case presentations can tell us whether students are thinking critically, solving problems, and expressing ideas clearly. Tape-recorded interviews can tell us more about communication skills than we can learn in our limited contact time with a student and patient.

Even now, in community health clinical courses, for example, instructors cannot always be present when students visit homes to give care. They may make two or three visits with each of their students, but in most cases they rely heavily on students' preplanning of the visit and postreporting of what actually happened during the visit. Community health nursing probably comes closest to process as content, since students are expected to learn what information they need and then to collect and use it.

Evaluation of Clinical Teaching Effectiveness

We have given a great deal of attention to evaluating what students do in the clinical area, but we have sorely neglected to evaluate clinical teaching methods in any systematic fashion. In their study of priority issues in nursing education research, Tanner and Lindeman (1987) found that whereas the first priority was the "integration of research findings from practice into the nursing curriculum" (p. 58), the second, third, and fourth priorities all were concerned with the development of problem-solving skills and the most effective approaches to clinical teaching. They concluded from the paucity of completed research studies that "there is little known about the effectiveness of approaches to clinical teaching in terms of student learning."

Infante (1975) points out that "nursing education has had an historical difficulty in identifying what clinical teaching consists of" (p. 17). McCabe (1985) calls "the improvement of instruction in the clinical area" a "challenge waiting to be met." She points out that whereas nurse educators are in agreement about the importance of clinical learning experiences, there is very little research to support the effectiveness of specific teaching behaviors. Several opinion samplings and mailed questionnaires about teacher characteristics and behavior have been reported, but the process itself has not been well explored, described, or tested.

Karuhije (1986) gathered data that support Carpenito and Duespohl's (1981) assertion that "most graduate programs do not provide individuals with basic information on clinical instruction" (p. ix). The great majority of respondents agreed with this statement and considered "clinical teaching strategies" the "most desired content item" (outranking evaluation of student performance!) in their graduate preparation as nurse educators.

Most nursing education programs require that faculty members have a master's degree in nursing as a teaching credential, but there is no corresponding requirement that they have formal preparation in clinical teaching, and many in fact have no such preparation. The reason is that such preparation is not easily available. And, we suggest, the reason why it is not available is that there is no existing body of research-supported knowledge defining just what clinical teaching behaviors are effective. We teach, therefore, as we have been taught, or perhaps as we wish we had been taught.

Surely, then, there is ample reason to consider changes in the way we assist students in their efforts to become what we are, to take our place, and to take the nursing profession well into the 21st century, as well as into the rest of this one.

REFERENCES

Benner, P. (1984). *From novice to expert*. Menlo Park, CA: Addison-Wesley.

Carpenito, L., & Duespohl, A. (1981). *A guide for effective clinical instruction*. Wakefield, MA: Nursing Resources.

Infante, M. S. (1975). *The clinical laboratory in nursing education*. New York: John Wiley & Sons.

Joel, L. A. (1987, September). The impact of DRGs on basic nursing education and curriculum implications. Paper prepared for the Mid-Atlantic Regional Nursing Association.

Karuhije, H. F. (1986). Educational preparation for clinical teachings: Perceptions of the nurse educator. *Journal of Professional Nursing, 25*(4), 137–143.

Matheney, R. V. (1969). Pre- and post-conferences for students. *American Journal of Nursing, 69*(2), 280–289.

McCabe, B. W. (1985). The improvement of instruction in the clinical area: A challenge waiting to be met. *Journal of Nursing Education, 24*(6), 255-257.

Phillips, S. J., & Kaempfer, S. H. (1987). Clinical teaching associate model: Implementation in a community hospital setting. *Journal of Professional Nursing, 3*(3), 165–175.

Primm, P. L. (1986). Entry into practice: Competency statements for BSNs and ADNs. *Nursing Outlook, 34*(3), 135–137.

Stull, M. K. (1986). Entry skills for BSNs. *Nursing Outlook, 34*(3), 138, 153.

Tanner, C. A., & Lindeman, C. A. (1987). Research in nursing education: Assumptions and priorities. *Journal of Nursing Education, 26*(2), 50–59.

Wolf, Z. R., & O'Driscoll, R. W. (1979). How useful is the preclinical conference? *Nursing Outlook, 27*(7), 455–457.

Woolley, A. S. (1985). Challenging RN students: Practicing assessment skills in an urban mission. *Nurse Educator, 10*(3), 32–33.

Woolley, A. S. (1977). The long and tortured history of clinical evaluation. *Nursing Outlook, 25*(5), 308–315.

7

Historical and Economic Perspectives on the Nursing Labor Force

Nancy P. Greenleaf

Deanne Bonnar (1985), Director for the Boston region of the Massachusetts Office for Children, says, in a paper on women's work:

> Throughout history, women have done most of the world's care-giving work, but their work has rarely entitled them to control resources in their own right. In order to survive, all societies must have systems for the production and care of the material basis of life, and for the reproduction and care of human life [itself]. (p. 67)

Economic systems as we know them have evolved in response to the production, exchange and maintenance of inanimate objects, what Bonnar means by the "material basis of life." People, on the other hand, are not "produced," but are brought about by a biological process called reproduction. The reproduction and maintenance (care) of people has traditionally taken place within the household or family and the work entailed therein performed by women as, in Hilary Graham's (1983) words, "A Labour of Love" (p.13).

This paper has three parts. Part one presents a discussion of the language and ideological implications of certain economic theories and concepts as they apply to the nursing workforce. Part two presents a picture of the growth and development of the nursing labor force in the United States throughout the 20th century. Part three reorients the discussion to the mission of nursing relative to the health care of the United States population with implications for nursing curricula.

ECONOMIC IDEAS AND BELIEFS

In *Economics in Perspective*, John Kenneth Galbraith (1987) puts forth a very readable critical history of economic thought in the western world. Consistent with his other writings, Galbraith gives a lucid description of how prevailing beliefs influence both the definition of value and the distribution of accumulated value. By pointing out the close relationship between belief and theory, he shows how powerful the language of theory has been in shaping and maintaining dominant ideology and how that ideology has in turn been used to serve the interests of dominant subgroups in societies. An example of this power of ideas may be seen in looking again at the above-cited passage about caregiving work. Since economic theories historically have dealt with the material basis of life, rather than life itself, the work involved in caring for life itself is totally absent from the analysis. Platitudes, such as "life is priceless," do little to soften the poverty of millions of women throughout the world whose life work is taking care of others.

Nonetheless, economic theories of value have persistently focused on the inanimate. According to Galbraith (1987), theories of value have varied over time but most have been concerned with the material resources required for producing things in combination with the labor required to transform raw materials into such things. The labor or work involved in reproducing and taking care of people themselves has not, until very recently, entered into discussions of value production. This would not be such a problem were it not that theories of value are so central to economic explanations used to inform and justify crucial policy decisions that effect our social resources.

Again according to Galbraith (1987), distribution, who gets what and why, is the second issue of economic theory. Around this issue gravitate the historical debates about communal versus private ownership of property. Of interest here, and as an example of the pervasiveness of the debate, are the differences of opinion held by Plato and his renowned pupil, Aristotle. Plato, it seems, conceived of a state where free enterprise prevailed among citizens (exclude women and slaves by definition). The rulers that guided and protected the state, however, would have to live ascetic lives renouncing private property beyond the barest essentials. If they became property owners, Plato feared they would become enemies of other citizens rather than proper guardians. Aristotle, on the other hand, was firmly in favor of the ownership of private property and of the pursuit of self-interest. For Aristotle, it was not the ownership per se, but the ethical relationship that the owner held toward his property, slaves, and women that counted.

Related to theories of distribution is the concept of the division of labor: who gets to do what. According to David Gil (1981), the distribution of work and the division of labor are not arbitrary or random: they are the result of policy decisions. Policies, Gil (1987) says, are rules that regularize human activity. He maintains that policies are made by people in charge and should not be credited or blamed on God. The acceptance of this premise begs the question of why caregiving work is so universally performed by women.

Caregiving Work as Economic Activity

The meaning of the concept "care" is so intertwined with nursing that the dictionary uses the phrase "in the care of a nurse" to illustrate the protective, supervisory connotation of the noun. The verb, to care, means to have a concern with or interest in the "other." To take care of a person, as opposed to an object, requires attention to the interest of that person. Attending to the interest of the other is antithetical to the idea of self-interest. The oppositional relationship of attending to the interest of the other and attending to the interest of the self is not unique to nursing and is evident in other service sector work. However, there can be little doubt that it can be derived directly from the definition of care of persons and that this in turn is a central component of the work of nursing.

Why is this important? Adam Smith, the 18th-century philosopher, broke important theoretical ground for economists by his assertion that the common good was best served by everyone acting in his own self-interest. Prior to Adam Smith, the idea of self-enrichment had been the object of much doubt and mistrust vis-à-vis the public interest. Smith's arguments in defense of self-interest turned an object of scorn into a public benefactor. It is not, however, this idea by itself, but its combination with Smith's metaphor of the invisible hand, that has so empowered dominant western ideology. In other words, if each person is allowed, without constraint, to pursue his own self-interest, such a free market will, like an invisible hand, assure the best outcome for all. The invisible hand metaphor takes on amazingly godlike qualities. Meanwhile, it sure is nice to have *some* people attending to the interests of others. Galbraith (1987) would call this "a convenient social virtue." It makes life easier for everyone, but clearly it is not what makes the world go around.

Another way of understanding this comes from the realization that nursing care must be given. Nurses give nursing care. They do not sell their nursing care, they sell their labor. Care, as in nursing care, requires a positive relational attitude that must be given. Nursing work is akin to what Bonnar (1987) means when she speaks of caregiving work. Nursing, it seems, is rooted in women's traditional role of a family caregiver that has historically remained outside of the market.

THE GROWTH AND DEVELOPMENT OF THE NURSING LABOR FORCE

The relationship between the industrialization of health care in the United States and the development of the nursing labor force is a familiar theme to students of nursing history. A particularly euphemistic reference to this relationship may be found in Paul Starr's (1982) Pulitzer Prize winner, *The Transformation of American Medicine*. Without mentioning nursing by name, Starr explains how physicians, unlike other artisans, were able to resist corporate domination and maintain the integrity of their craft as well as the control over the division of labor of less skilled but essential aides. Starr says:

> Doctors did not simply want to maintain a "monopoly of competence." They wanted to be able to use hospitals and laboratories without being their employees, and consequently they needed technical assistants who would be sufficiently competent to carry on in their absence and yet not threaten their authority. The solution to this problem—how to maintain autonomy, yet not lose control—had three elements: first, the use of doctors in training in the operation of hospitals; second, the encouragement of a kind of responsible professionalism among the higher ranks of subordinate health workers; and third, the employment in these auxiliary roles of women who, though professionally trained, would not challenge the authority or economic position of the doctor. (pp. 220–221)

Starr thus demonstrates a critical economic difference between medicine, as practiced by physicians, and nursing, as practiced by professional nurses, in the former's ability to resist becoming a wage worker, by making use of the highly skilled services of the latter.

Nursing's history is very different. It is helpful to the understanding of the role of nurse as employee to look at how reports of nursing shortages over time have shaped the development of the nursing labor force as we know it today.

The Nursing Shortages of the 20th Century

For the greater part of the 20th century there have been claims (Yett, 1975) of insufficient nursing personnel to adequately staff hospitals in the United States. These claims have varied from overall shortages to inadequate skill mix or geographical maldistribution. Responses to these claims have, for the most part, aimed at increasing the supply of nurses primarily through government subsidization of education. Issues of nursing shortage are rarely discussed by policymakers in the context of the health status of the American people and their needs for nursing services. Rather, the nursing labor force has been analyzed from the point of view of the needs of the health care industry. Historically, concerns about nursing shortages have been most acute when hospitals have been forced to close beds for lack of sufficient personnel. Indeed, the nursing shortage is usually operationally defined as the number of unfilled positions reported by the industry.

Another fact often ignored in discussions of nursing labor shortages is their relationship to the overall economy. There have always been more nurses available for work during economic downturns. In the years of the Great Depression there are reports that nurses offered their services to hospitals in exchange for room and board. More recently, amidst the 1982 recession, the *Wall Street Journal*'s Labor Letter reported: " . . . nurse shortage eases in some areas, partly because of the recession." In times of high economic growth however, Yett (1975) and Lublin (1980) reported significant increases in vacancy rates.

Reports of nursing shortages have persisted throughout most of this century, even though the production of nursing school graduates has steadily increased. Figure 1 shows the number of active registered nurses and practicing physicians for selected times thoughout the century. "Active registered" here means currently licensed but not necessarily employed.

In the early part of the century, the growth of hospitals and of nursing schools went hand in hand, with student nurses providing most of the hospital labor force. There were few controls, educational or otherwise, on the production of nurses. For instance, a detailed study (Drew, 1985) of the industry growth in Maine over the last century demon-

Figure 1
Historical Data on Nurse & Physician Supply in U.S.

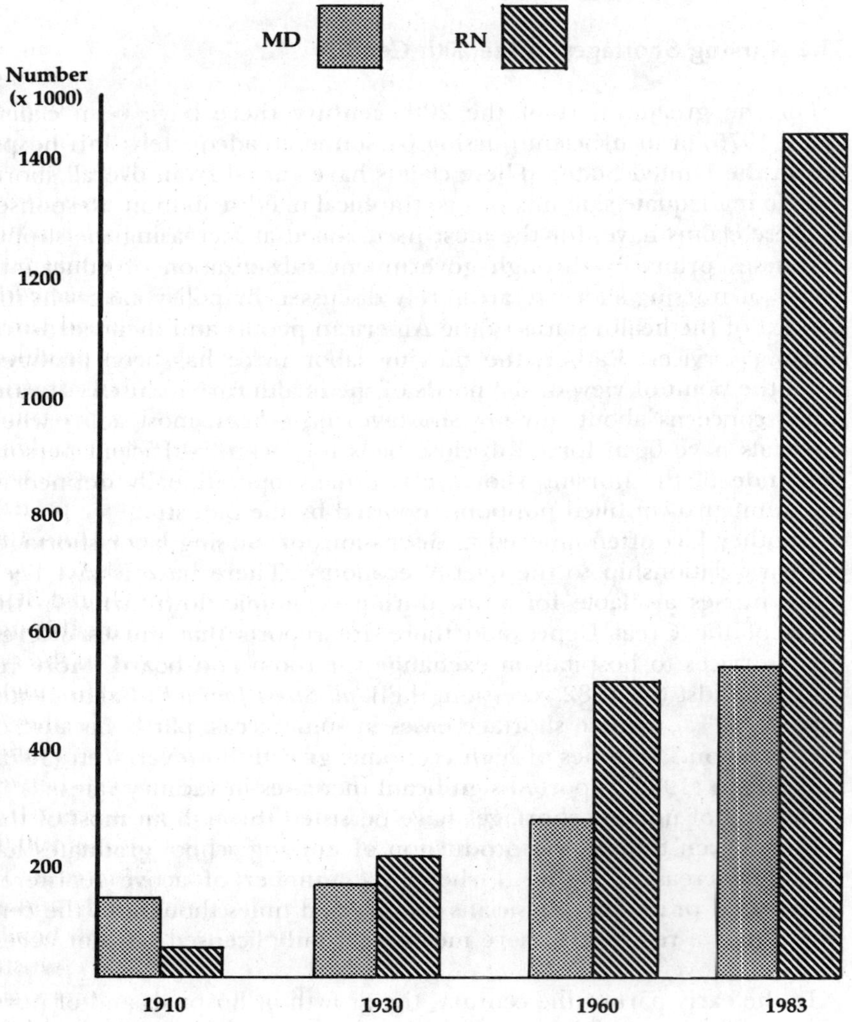

Source: Bureau of the Census: Historical Statistics of the United States (Figures on physicians and nurses, 1910–1963): Series B, 275–290.

Bureau of the Census: Statistical Abstract of the United States (Figures on physicians and nurses, 1983): Series B, 275–290.

strates that many hospital-based nursing schools had more student nurses than patients. By the late 1920s, there was great concern expressed from within the profession (Burgess, 1928) over the excess numbers of graduates who were having difficulty finding employment. During the 1930s, this labor surplus gradually dissipated and by the onset of World War II nursing shortages were being reported in all sections of the country. The growth of the nurse supply continued through midcentury (Yett, 1975) fueled by the labor mobilization of the Second World War, the post-war hospital construction boom, and continuing reports of shortages.

In spite of this rapid growth in the nurse supply, by the early 1960s the vacancy rate for full-time hospital positions for RNs had reached over 20 percent. As reported by Yett (1975), one in five hospital positions went unfilled. In 1964, the Nurse Training Act (NTA) enacted by Congress initiated a 298 million dollar program which it hoped would lead to a 75 percent increase in the annual number of nurses produced by 1975. The NTA included authorization for nursing school construction, grants to schools to expand and strengthen teaching programs, grants to hospital schools to help offset the costs of additional students, traineeships to fund graduate education for nurses to become teachers, administrators, supervisors and specialists, and low-interest, partially forgivable loans. The dramatic increase in the nurse supply from 1960 through the early 1980s is largely due to this Congressional Act.

Figure 2 depicts trends in the rates per 100,000 of the United States population of hospital beds, registered nurses, and physicians throughout the century. Aggregate data such as these cannot speak to the type of work nurses engage in, geographical distribution or technological changes that affect the work process. However, neither can they be ignored. The picture is dramatic, particularly the changing relationships between the rates for registered nurses and hospital beds between 1960 and the early 1980s. As hospital beds declined 19 percent from 1,658,000 in 1960 to 1,350,000 in 1983, the rate of nurses per 100,000 of the population went from 148 to 228, a 179 percent increase. The changing relationship between the number of hospital beds and the nurse supply forces us to ask more pointedly: how have the benefits of the nurse supply been distributed? Figures for 1985 (Statistical Abstract of the United States [SAUS], 1987, p.91) show there were 1,447,000 employed nurses in the United States. With a United States population for that year of 239,238,000 (Statistical Abstract of the United States, p.8), we had one employed registered nurse for every 165 Americans. Surely our population is not so moribund. These fig-

Figure 2
Historical Data: Rates per 100,000 of population for

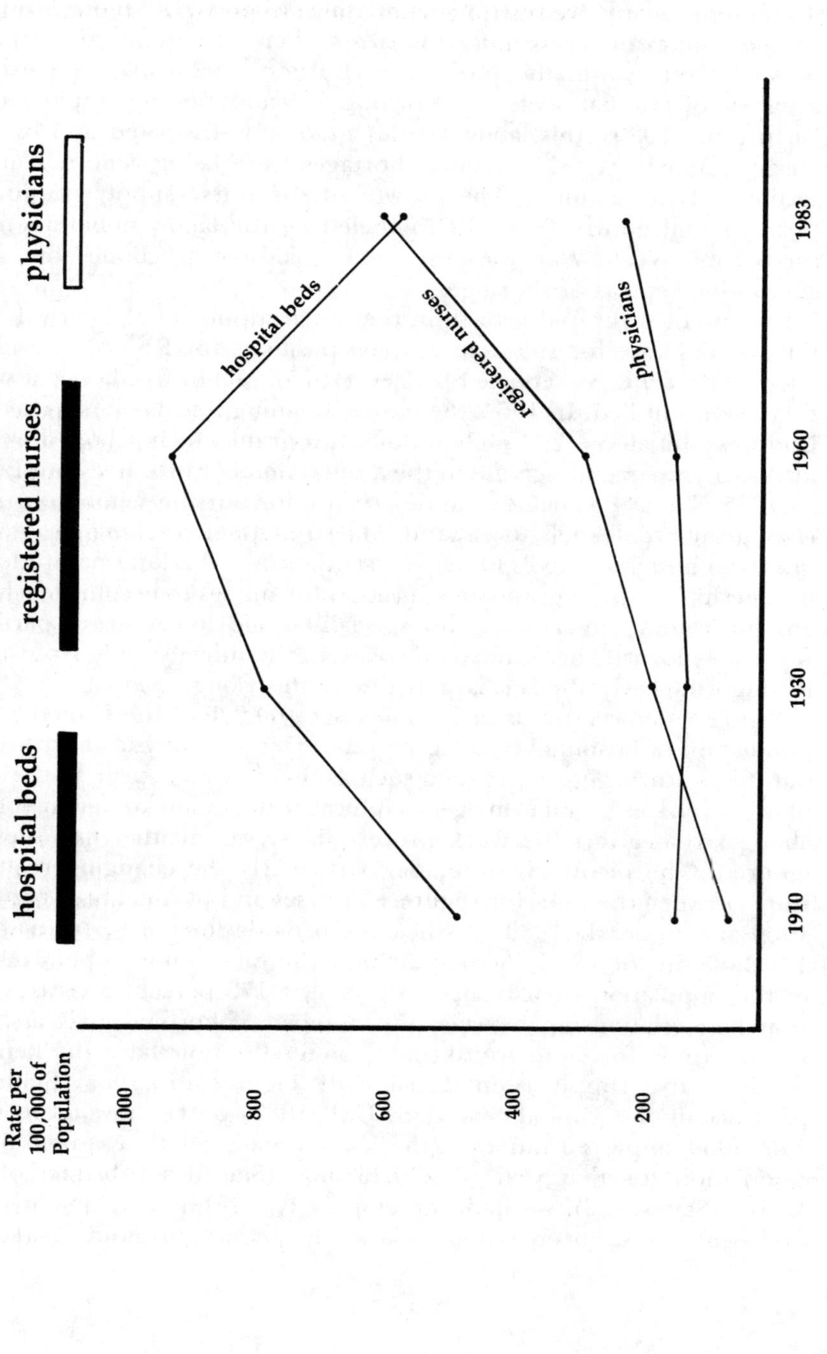

Source: Bureau of the Census: Historical Statistics of the United States.

ures become even more startling when they are juxtaposed to information about people's access to health care.

NURSING AND HEALTH

Before looking at the health of the people of the United States, it serves our purpose to think for a moment about the mission of nursing. As nursing knowledge has progressed during the recent past, intellectual work has focused on theory and its explications. Chinn and Jacobs (1983) have proposed a quite acceptable definition of theory as "a systematic abstraction of reality that serves some purpose" (p. 2). It is this purpose, or mission of nursing that must be considered when curricula are evaluated. Benner (1984) suggests a primary purpose of nursing when she uses "significant contribution to a patient's (other's) welfare" (p. xviii), in describing her selection of nursing exemplars. Indeed, attending to the promotion, restoration, and maintenance of people's health has traditionally defined the purpose, or mission of nursing.

How well then is the nursing workforce positioned to fulfill this mission? How is it that people, whose health care requires nurses, gain access to nursing care? What are the economic forces that impact on the distribution of nursing care?

Poverty and the Need for Caring

There is little doubt in the minds of most students of the subject that poverty and poor health are related. Figure 3 shows that the proportion of people reporting fair to poor health goes from 4.6 percent for those with incomes over $35,000 to 21.1 percent for people with incomes under $10,000. Not surprisingly, the number of bed disability days per year for people with incomes under $5,000 is three times higher than for people with incomes over $25,000. Figure 4 shows that of poor people reporting fair to poor health, blacks outnumber whites by 10 percentage points.

In Figure 5, by looking at increasing inequality we can see that the distance between the rich and the poor is widening. If we look at the experience of other countries, where the rich and the poor are separated by wide gaps, we will see that the health care available to the poorer sectors of society is meager. Figure 6 shows a further breakdown of the poverty level of families by the gender of family head and

Figure 3
Percent of Population in Fair or Poor Health by Family Income

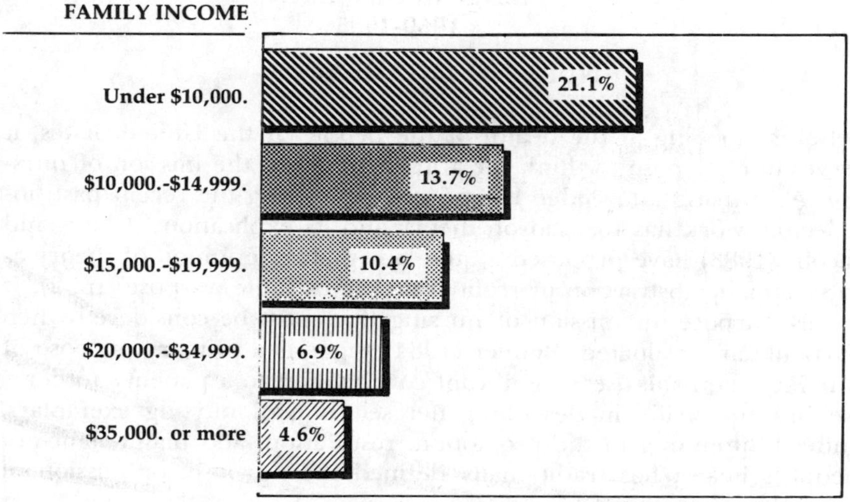

Source: Division of Health Interview Statistics, National Center for Health Statistics: Data from the National Health Interview Survey.

Figure 4
Percent of Population in Fair or Poor Health

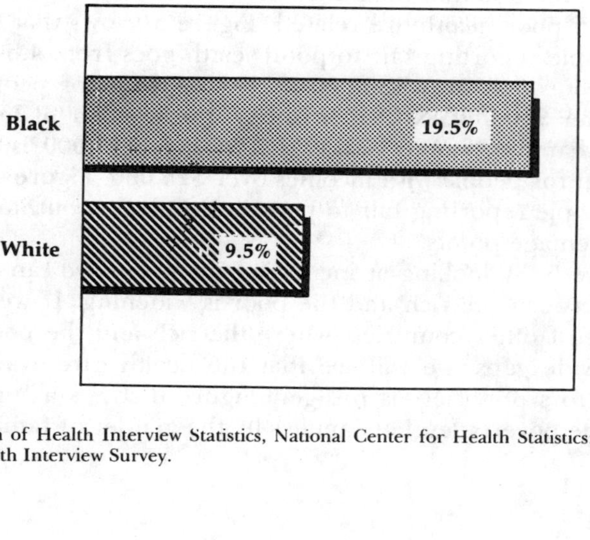

Source: Division of Health Interview Statistics, National Center for Health Statistics: Data from the National Health Interview Survey.

Figure 5
Surge in Inequality
1960-1985

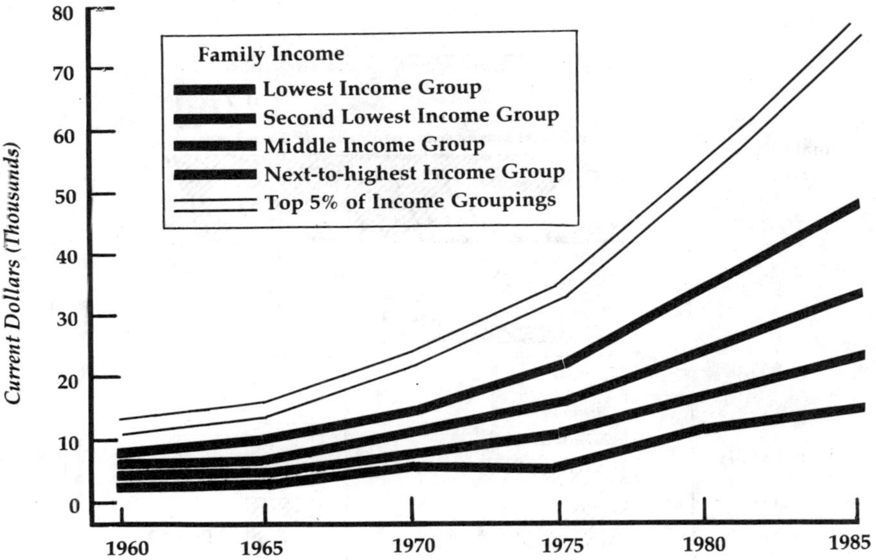

Source: Thurow, L.C. (1987) A surge in inequality. *Scientific American, 256*(5):30–37.

race. Clearly the largest shift is between male- and female-headed families for all races. Figure 7 shows the percentage below the poverty level by both age and race. Children are, as you see, abundant among the poor. As the gap between the rich and the poor widens, women, children, and nonwhites are overrepresented in the poverty group.

Poverty goes hand in hand with lack of the basic necessities of food and shelter which further undermines the health of many Americans. It is estimated that 20 million people in this country are hungry; that is, short of sufficient nutrients to sustain proper growth and good health. This growing problem, as reported by Brown (1987), is not surprising considering that $7 billion was transferred away from the food stamp program and another $5 billion was transferred away from the child nutrition program between 1982 and 1985.

The homeless population in the United States, as reported by Rossi, Wright, Fisher, and Willis (1987), is now estimated to be anywhere

Figure 6
Percent Below Poverty Level of Families by Sex of Family Head and Race

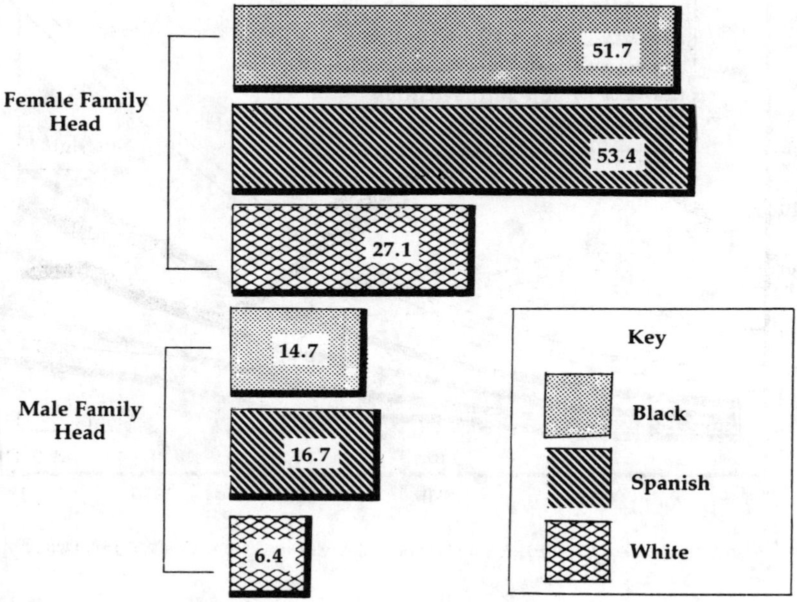

Source: Bureau of the Census: Current Population Reports. Series P-60, No. 149, Page 26.

from a quarter of a million to 3 million. Many of these people have moderate to severe health problems as any of the volunteers who staff shelters for the homeless can attest. For the hungry and homeless, lack of access to adequate nursing care is but one of a number of deprivations to endure.

The Distribution of Health and Nursing Care

Access to health care in the United States has been traditionally understood as access to physicians for diagnosis, and, where necessary, to hospitals or other agencies for treatment. Insurance, which has been of

Figure 7
Percent of Persons Below Poverty Level By Age & Race

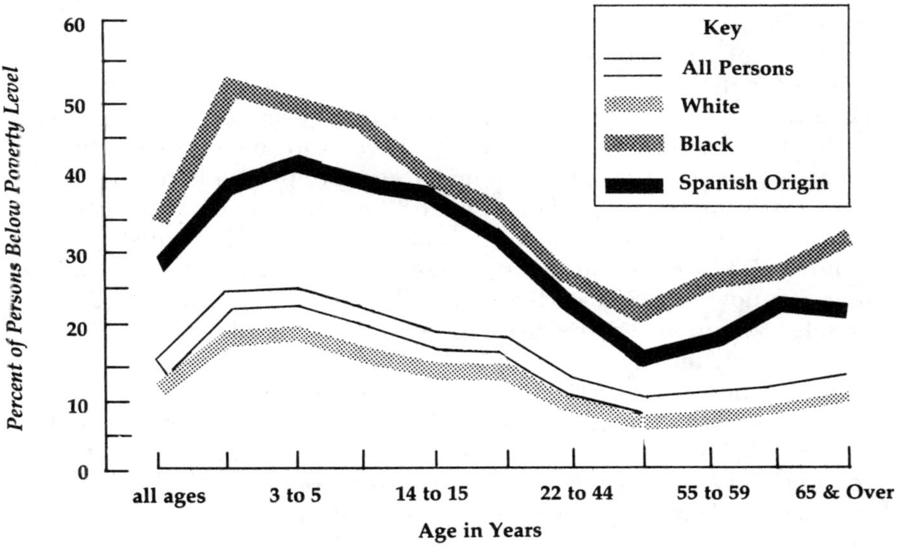

Source: Bureau of the Census: Current Population Reports. Series P-60, No. 149, Page 26.

vital importance to the development of the health care industry, has the effect of socializing the cost risk for both physician and hospital services. With the advent of federally funded Medicare and Medicaid programs, virtually all physician and hospital fees should be reimbursed by third-party payers. However, a recent American Hospital Association (1986) study has found that at any given time 13 to 16 percent of the United States population lack any health insurance coverage and another 10 percent have inadequate or unreliable coverage. According to the American Hospital Association (1986), together this accounts for at least 40 million Americans who are denied access to existing hospital services. Most of the uninsured are both employed and poor. They are simply not covered by either private or public insurance. Therefore, since only physicians can admit people to the health care agencies where nurses are employed and since some type of insurance coverage is usually a requirement for routine admissions, it is clear that access to nursing care is controlled by access to physicians and insurance.

More recently, cost containment efforts aimed at controlling inflation in health care are further eroding people's access to nursing care. The early discharge decision leads to a sicker patient mix in hospitals, a situation that requires more (not less) highly skilled nurses. Further, patients are often discharged before they are ready to assume full responsibility for their own care from a nursing point of view. The increased need for home nursing care is therefore quite common. Yet the refusal of Medicare to reimburse home health visits to these patients further restricts people's access to nursing care. Attempts made to have families absorb the work involved in taking care of patients who have been discharged early counts on each family having an able-bodied member at home. This policy fails because most "able-bodied" women as well as men are now in the labor force. The "family" is not at home. Forcing people to drop out of the labor force to take care of sick family members will only increase poverty.

At the most fundamental level then, we must acknowledge that the nursing workforce is not positioned in such a way that the mission of nursing can be fulfilled for a good many Americans. One employed registered nurse for every 165 Americans is not enough! If we subtract the medically indigent, whose access to health care institutions and thus to nursing care is severely limited, we will have one employed nurse for every 138 Americans. We may well ask in what activity are these nurses employed? Whose interest does their employment serve?

CONCLUSION

In an essay on humanistic education, Freire (1985) contrasts humanistic education with dehumanization. He says:

> Dehumanization is a concrete expression of alienation and domination; humanistic education is a utopian project of the dominated and the oppressed. Obviously both imply action by people in a social reality—the first, in the sense of preserving the status quo, the second in a radical transformation of the oppressor's world. (p. 113)

Similarly, we could contrast caring and its opposite, neglecting. Both caring and neglecting imply action in a social reality. Caring is a primary purpose of nursing, neglecting is a thwarting of that purpose. We cannot do both, we must choose. We cannot, in nursing, implement curricula that promote caring behaviors and, at the same time, claim neutrality toward access to care. It is antithetical to the mission of nursing to accept the neglect of certain subgroups.

I would suggest that we already have in place concepts and traditions that take us in directions consistent with nursing's mission. We teach change theory and practice. The subtitle of this conference is "Mandate for Change." Economic forces are historically marshalled to the service of dominant groups of the population. These economic forces have indeed played a major role in the positioning of the nursing workforce vis-à-vis the care of people. In nursing, we must broaden our analysis and use of change theory and practice and challenge economic structures that deny certain subgroups access to nursing care. This cannot happen without courage. It is not accidental that things are as they are.

REFERENCES

American Hospital Association. (1986). *Cost and compassion: Recommendations for avoiding a crisis in care for the medically indigent.* Chicago: Author.

Benner, P. (1984). *From novice to expert: Excellence and power in clinical nursing practice.* Menlo Park, CA: Addison-Wesley.

Bonnar, D. (1987). Women, work and poverty: Exit from an ancient trap by the redefinition of work. In D. G. Gil & E. A. Gil (Eds.), *The Future of Work.* Cambridge, MA: Shenkman.

Brown, L. (1987, February). Hunger in the U.S. *Scientific American,* 256:2.

Burgess, M.A. (1928). *Nurses patients and pocketbooks.* New York: The Committee on the Grading of Nursing Schools.

Chinn, P., & Jacobs, M. K. (1983). *Theory and nursing: A systematic approach.* St. Louis: C.V. Mosby.

Drew, J. (1985, May). *Nursing schools in Maine—1900 to 1985.* Paper presented at the University of Maine, Presque Isle, ME.

Freire, P. (1985). *The politics of education: Culture, power and liberation.* Massachusetts: Bergin and Garvey.

Galbraith, J. K. (1987). *Economics in perspective: A critical history.* Boston: Houghton Mifflin.

Gil, D. G. (1981). *Unraveling social policy.* (3rd ed.). Cambridge, MA: Shenkman.

Gil, D. G. (1987, April). *Lecture on social policy.* Unpublished manuscript, University of Southern Maine, School of Nursing, Portland, ME.

Graham, H. (1983). Caring: A labour of love. In J. Finch & D. Groves (Eds.), *A Labour of Love: Women, Work and Caring.* London: Routledge and Kegan Paul.

Lubin, J. S. (1980). Critical condition: Severe nurse shortage forces some hospitals to close beds or units. *The Wall Street Journal*, p. 1, 9.

Rossi, P., Wright, J. D., Fisher, G. A., & Willis, G. (1987, March 13). The urban homeless: Estimating composition and size. *Science*, 231.

Starr, P. (1982). *The social transformation of American medicine*. New York: Basic Books.

Thurow, L. C. (1987). A surge in inequality. *Scientific Americare*, *256*(5):30–37.

Yett, D. E. (1975). *An economic analysis of the nursing shortage*. Lexington, MA: D.C. Heath.

8

Curriculum Revolution: A Bioethical Mandate for Change

Mila Ann Aroskar

> Nurses . . . and others are often insufficiently prepared to deal responsibly with the choices technology requires. This raises ethical questions about the obligations of educational programs to prepare students for such environments. Education for the health professions which does not include consideration of ethical issues related to technology is inadequate and irresponsible. (Aroskar, 1987, p. 15)

As these statements suggest, I believe that a curriculum revolution in nursing is urgently needed. If we are to make the best possible choices about the use of technology in nursing and health care, we must develop new paradigms that will help us to teach and learn how to make better decisions in patient/client care and in policy-making situations complicated by moral conflict. This is part of the broader realm of clinical judgment. Technology is not just the invention and use of machines, drugs, or procedures; it is also any systematic, disciplined approach to achieving objectives or any organized means of affecting the social or physical environment. In this latter sense, it can refer both to development of knowledge (research) and use of that knowledge in dealing with practical tasks and problems. Use of the nursing process, then, can be considered a technology.

Nurses, who often find themselves caught in the middle between patients, physicians, families, and administrators, face a wide variety of situations involving use of technology at different levels. They must make difficult choices about treatment, and often no ready-made answers are available to them. Nurses are required to create ethically adequate responses in such situations, that is, responses that take into account the ethical dimensions of their decision making. They are moral agents who take on considerable responsibility for the safety and well-being of clients but whose authority or power is often insufficiently recognized. In order to teach students to fill such a position in health care organizations, we as nurse educators must look carefully at several challenges to nursing curricula that have recently been raised. In part, these challenges arise from new kinds of moral conflict in health care that have been generated by use of technology. Moral and philosophical concerns, such as autonomy, behavior control, promise keeping, avoiding or preventing harm, paternalism or parentalism, personhood, beneficence, and justice in health care are not unique to nurses. What is unique is the place of nurses and nursing in health care organizations, the nature of nursing knowledge, and the perspective and expertise shared by most nurses, which influence whether and how nurses deal with ethical challenges in their daily practice.

MORAL CENTRALITY OF NURSING

The philosopher and ethicist Andrew Jameton (1984) asserts that "nursing is the morally central health care profession" (p.xvi). He argues that the values and principles most closely associated with nursing—that is, compassion and health—are the values that should guide health care practice. He also believes that clinical practice would pose fewer ethical dilemmas and benefit patients more if nurses directed health care practice more actively and received more recognition for their professional viewpoint. Many of us would agree; however, we would also agree that philosophical approaches to moral problems in clinical settings are of limited usefulness to nurses. To diminish the moral conflicts nurses now face—such as feelings of obligation to clients created by the nursing shortage and cost-containment efforts—social and organizational changes are necessary. This suggests that there is a mandate not only for change in how ethics are taught but also for greater sensitivity to the politics and economics of practicing ethics in the muddy waters where money and power count.

If Jameton is correct, the burden on nurse educators and systems of nursing education is perhaps greater than has been recognized either by the profession itself or by decision makers in health care systems external to nursing. To develop and implement curricula that are adequate to today's challenges, nothing short of a revolution—that is, a radical and fundamental change—is required. This was recognized a decade ago by Churchill (1977), who argues that professions in transition, such as nursing, need to develop critical self-awareness and to keep asking themselves what they are and what they should be (which are questions of ethics). Churchill believes that the training for health professions, in this instance nursing, should have two fundamental working ethics. One is an ethic of *competence*, that is, being good at what one does and performing according to the standards of the profession. This is an internally driven professional ethic. The second is an ethic of *compassion* or, alternatively, an ethic of *caring*. This ethic is more patient driven, and requires nurses to practice with understanding and empathy. This ethic is grounded in a sense of the shared humanity of both patients and caregivers and is expressed in the felt needs and values lived by nurses and their patients/clients. Such an ethic requires attention to the humanity of nursing students and clients in planning the curriculum.

Churchill (1977) goes on to suggest that the ethic of competence should be responsive to an ethic of compassion as the motivating force of the nursing profession. In fact, however, most nursing curricula, like the curricula of other health professions, focus primarily on competence and only secondarily on compassion. This may put health professionals, including nurses, at a disadvantage in the process of self-examination, and it may obscure their sense of obligation to the individuals, groups, or communities they profess to serve. Churchill's comments point to what could and should be a revolutionary and fundamental change in nursing curricula, one that goes beyond the present accreditation criteria (which include ethics only as one item in a list).

In recent times, some nursing curricula have placed great emphasis on fostering a sense of "community." Let us ask ourselves, what would health care be like if compassion and caring were the major grounding concepts for nursing curricula, and the major goal for nursing and health care systems was the creation of caring, compassionate communities that took seriously the welfare and humanity of both clients and caregivers? Certainly it would be very different from health care today, in which the focus is most often on use of the latest technologies, competition, cost containment or shifting, and dealing with the nursing shortage. Though such idealistic visions are not likely to be realized tomorrow or the day after, they are still worth considering; in fact, they have already received concerted attention in the work of nursing leaders such as Carper, Watson, and Leininger. Pursuit of such goals and ideals in nursing curricula is a far more radical step than the simple introduction of an ethics course into the curriculum. It argues for curricula that deal with the realms of technological meaning, politics, and ethics. Ethics and politics overlap in the worlds of nursing practice, for they both address conflicts of needs and interests between individuals and groups, and they both dwell at the interface between ethical responsibility and power.

Key elements to take in to account when considering curriculum changes are the nurse-patient-technology relationship and the overlap of ethics and politics in the practice of applied and professional ethics in nursing and health care. A good deal of attention has been paid to the nurse-patient relationship and the light that nursing theories and work in nursing ethics shed on this relationship. Much less attention has been paid to the nurse-patient-technology relationship. In the late 20th century, it is impossible to fully understand the nurse-patient or nurse-physician relationship without understanding the use and meaning of technology in this context.

THE TECHNOLOGICAL CONTEXT

In a recent work, political scientist Langdon Winner (1986) explores the relationship between technologies and how we live and work. He argues that the kind of technologies we build and use represent choices about who we want to be and what kind of world we want to create, and he believes that we are "sleepwalking" through the process of reconstituting the very conditions of our existence. He claims that decisions about development of technologies are not only technical decisions but also *political* decisions about power, liberty, social order, and justice. Automation of industries and wide use of computers are examples of technopolitical systems that represent choices about who we want to be and about what kind of world we want to create. If Winner's perceptions and arguments are accurate, we must seriously consider some combined practice that takes into account the connections among ethics, politics, and technology in all our social systems, including nursing and health care.

It is obvious that we are in fact reconstituting the conditions of nursing and health care in the latter part of the 20th century. Technologies such as kidney dialysis, transplantation, and use of mechanical respirators are not merely aids to human activity: they are also powerful forms that reshape our activities and their meanings, as well as powerful symbols of the power to save life and the power to torment life. In addition, we, as a society, are creating population groups—such as ventilator-dependent patients and transplant patients—who must remain on complex treatment regimens for the rest of their lives. Reiser and Anbar (1984) remind us that technology helps us to improve patient quality of life, but it also allows us to sustain life under conditions of great suffering. We can use technology to perform life-saving miracles, or we can use it to prolong suffering and dying.

TECHNOLOGY IN NURSING CARE

Nurses' responsibilities and obligations to patients are greatly influenced by technology. Use of computers in patient care, for example, increases nurses' responsibilities for developing and interpreting the clinical data base to patients. These responsibilities are at the interface between human and nonhuman elements. As practitioners who use machines, nurses must be careful never to avoid responsibility for consequences of their use. Reiser and Anbar (1984) warn us that machines can make us forget ourselves, because to a greater or lesser extent they establish a "technological buffer" between patients and caregivers. In this view, the human-machine interface does jeopardize the human component of health care. For example, the stress of attempting to maintain the technologies of patient care has the potential to blunt the emotional commitment of caregivers to patient care.

My attention was first drawn to the nurse-patient-machine triad in a coronary intensive care unit a few years ago. Each patient was in a separate room, and all the doors were closed. The nurses were sitting in the nurses' station observing the machines. One of them, on leaving for a coffee break, said to the other, "Take care of the machines while I'm gone." I wondered then if the nurses were treating human responses or mechanical responses. More than one nurse has complained about having to nurse machines instead of patients. Smith and Brdlik (1985) quote Lenihan and Abbey as stating that

> nurses nurse machines when they lack information about the instrument and how it functions, what its capabilities are, where the limits are, when it can be hazardous, and why it is being used. In this instance, largely because of ignorance, the instrument ceases to be a clinical tool by which a nurse can obtain reliable physiologic in-

> formation, and becomes a totem with dials, beeps, and lights that can scream false alarm when electrodes are crossed. (p.1)

If use of machines (and other technologies) in patient care does indeed influence nurse-patient relationships and, consequently, the nature of patient care and decision making (as I believe it does), this must be taken into account in the planning of curricula.

According to Reiser and Anbar (1984), how to marshall technology and people to meet the needs of an individual patient efficiently and humanely is a central problem of modern health care. They assert that the triadic relationship between practitioners, patients, and machines is one of the most difficult of associations to master. Such concerns present a challenge to those of us who make decisions about nursing curricula and research in nursing education. They challenge our concepts of advocacy and caring, challenge the humanity and integrity of nurses and the nursing profession, challenge nursing leaders, and challenge the structures and organizations within which nursing care is delivered.

Nursing has already made some progress toward considering the implications of the use of technology in health care; it has recognized that nurses are in an excellent position to raise questions, to monitor the uses of technology in patient care, and to provide the dimension of compassion that is required in dealing with human responses to health problems. In addition, both nurses and physicians recognize that how humans react to machines and technology can be and often is as important a factor in treatment as the disease itself. As advocates, nurses are obliged to understand how use of technology affects the nurse-client relationship, how to integrate serious consideration of patient responses into the determination of whether use of technology enhances patient welfare and autonomy, and how to develop ethically sensitive nursing interventions for those responses. As advocates, nurses are in an excellent position to ensure that the patients' voices are heard in decision making when there are disagreements about treatment decisions, when patients suffer from a feeling of loss of control, or when treatments are adding to rather than decreasing patient suffering.

How can we teach so as to ensure that students learn about their rights, obligations, and commitments to patients and clients in technologically complex and stressful environments? A first step might be to reverse our current ethical priorities. The ethic of competence seemingly has been taking and continues to take precedence in nursing curricula; however, we must recognize that an ethic of competence can only be based on an ethic of compassion.

IMPLICATIONS FOR CURRICULUM

The literature on nurses' moral development and moral reasoning is growing rapidly. From the literature, we know that education affects nurses' responses to ethical problems, at least in an academic sense. Nursing researchers are still studying the links between moral reasoning and clinical judgment in nursing: in the meantime, I offer a few ideas for nursing education experiences in applied ethics that may prove useful. I begin with what I consider to be a seminal case study of high technology in patient care (Schucking, 1985). This case study could be used by schools of nursing in entry-level, master's, and doctoral programs. It has the added benefit of including comments from experts in nursing, medicine, law, and hospital administration. I follow it with some descriptive research that may yield clues to potential avenues for curricular reform.

Case Study

Brenda Hewitt, a 53-year-old editor and poet, died in a prestigious New York hospital after eight years of suffering from kidney disease that developed as a complication of diabetes. She experienced "almost continuous, unimaginable pain," according to the person who chronicled her death, a physics professor and the man who loved and cared for her during those eight years (Schucking, 1985). She died in a critical care unit, surrounded by and subjected to the most sophisticated technologies available, including full resuscitation, which she had specifically rejected in the handwritten notarized advance directive ("living will") she had drawn up with the help of an attorney. In a painful account of her last hours at home and in a critical care unit, Schucking describes his frustrated efforts to make the medical staff take Brenda Hewitt's wishes and values into account as they formulated their numerous treatment decisions. Some of those decisions, such as the decision to try resuscitation and mechanical respiration—which she specifically rejected in her living will—were clearly of no medical benefit to her and in fact only added to her suffering.

There is no evidence of any meaningful nursing intervention on Brenda Hewitt's behalf, no sign of any nursing support for the author, who was the person she authorized to speak for her, and no mention of any meaningful nursing care. Two nurses' aides appear in the account: one tried to remove the author from Ms. Hewitt's bedside, and the other came only to take away the television. The conclusion I can reach from Schucking's account of Ms. Hewitt's death is that the most basic nursing care needs received little or no attention. One could, of course, argue that this disturbing account of one patient's treatment may be an anomaly, and that it should be balanced against the positive accounts of nursing care that have been recorded in many institutions. Still, however, Brenda Hewitt's case raises deeply troubling questions, questions that must be faced by the nursing profession, as a collective body of practitioners with an implicit social contract to provide competent humane nursing care, by individual nurses, who express or negate this contract in practice, and certainly by nurse educators.

Brenda Hewitt expressed her wishes clearly and unambiguously, but those wishes were ignored. The available technologies were inappropriately used to sustain her life when she no longer wanted to live. According to one physician, who disregarded the patient's instructions, the medical staff was "erring on the side of life." In this instance, availability of technology dominated decision making. Schools of nursing could use this case study (with different objectives) as a common link for students in entry-level, master's, and doctoral programs. Because it also includes commentary from professionals in other disciplines, it could be used for multidisciplinary study as well.

Objectives

The literature supplies many possible objectives for the teaching of ethics in nursing. In entry-level programs, an overall objective might be to develop students' ability to practice nursing in ethically sensitive ways which enhance rather than detract from holistic patient/client care. Another objective might be to prepare student nurses to participate actively at the patient care and institutional level in ethics rounds and in nursing and biomedical ethics committees. If Jameton's (1984) contention that nursing's values are morally central to health care is correct, then we must find curricular means to promote these values more explicitly. To achieve this goal, we must ensure that faculty members pay attention not only to teaching skills of ethical reasoning but also to alleviating those conditions in the practice setting that impede ethically sensitive practice and resolution of moral conflict. The ANA (1985) explicitly outlines the responsibility of nurse educators in this area.

In undergraduate programs, educators could use Schucking's account of Brenda Hewitt's death in teaching students to identify ethical issues and concerns, to examine ethical principles such as autonomy and beneficence, and to consider the issues from the perspective of ethical theory. In this way, they might be able to impart a more vivid vision of more ethically adequate systems of health care that take into account both clients and caregivers. In some nursing curricula, learning opportunities of this sort are planned for in class and clinical settings.

In graduate programs, students could reexamine the same case study with an eye to exploring concepts of personhood and management/administrative issues. The latter are often issues of distributive justice, involving as they do the equitable distribution of benefits and burdens in nursing and health care. One example is the allocation of the scarce resource of nursing expertise within institutions in the present environment of shortage, cost shifting, and competition. Although issues of justice may seem distant to nurses, they directly and indirectly affect the care that nurses provide. Such issues also underlie the decisions made by individual nurses about how to allocate time to patients and the decisions made by nurse executives about how to allocate nursing staff with particular kinds of expertise to ensure safe care throughout their institutions. Study of Brenda Hewitt's case will encourage many students to ask questions about the fair and ethically adequate allocation of nursing expertise, as well as about other ethical concerns, such as autonomy and nonmaleficence (avoiding or preventing harm).

Faced with situations where distributive justice and nurses' fidelity to patients are at issue, some nurses, and perhaps some students, ask themselves whether they really want to remain in nursing when they are unable to provide safe and competent care because of institutional or societal constraints. In such circumstances, nurses may feel that they are working in an "ethical wasteland." It is therefore essential that nurses in graduate programs have opportunities to consider their obligations to develop and maintain high-quality, morally adequate systems of nursing care, in which nurses do not feel totally frustrated and damaged as moral agents. Failure to provide these opportunities may give rise to the evil the philosopher Nel Noddings (1984) warns of:

> There can be no greater evil, then, than this: that the moral autonomy of the one caring be so shattered that she acts against her own commitment to care. (p.115)

From Noddings's perspective, failure to care puts the individual's very integrity and wholeness at stake—a critical consideration for nursing education.

Obviously, nursing educators cannot create new systems of care by themselves. For significant improvements in the quality of patient care, collective action by nurses and the nursing profession that explicitly takes account of ethical principles and values is required. Fry (1982) notes this in her discussion of the place of the clinical laboratory in teaching and in the development of morally adequate systems of care. Fry regards attention to ethical principles and value orientations as the missing link between education and practice. One hopes that Brenda Hewitt would have been treated differently if she had been under the care of ethically and politically sensitive nurses who were aware of their responsibilities as client advocates.

A final note about Brenda Hewitt's case: faculty should be aware of both the strengths and the limitations of case studies. Among their strengths are that they ground analysis and inquiry in practice situations that are more compelling than abstractions, that they help students to move more easily between the concrete and the abstract, and that they demonstrate the need for interdisciplinary contributions in gathering "facts" such as legal, medical, and social information. Among their limitations are that when sufficient time for presentation and discussion is lacking (which is usually the case), participants frequently do not progress beyond trying to determine what information they need to reach a decision. (I call this the "wow, what a case" limitation.) It is sometimes difficult to move into more abstract areas of ethical discussion; there is a tendency to move from identifying issues and data needed directly to making decisions for action. This may be because much education in the health professions, including nursing, focuses on the presentation of information and the use of objective tests for evaluation rather than on providing learning situations that require students to think critically and reflectively and then to make decisions on the basis of those reflections.

As a result, many students have had no experience with basic philosophical approaches to issues and problems. Such approaches must be incorporated into nursing curricula, either as prerequisites or as a sequence of learning opportunities. An additional concern is that health care professionals, most of whom are action-oriented problem solvers, have a tendency to look for ready-made solutions (the "just tell me what to do" limitation). Consequently, they are easily frustrated when lengthy discussion does not lead to a definite "answer" that tells them what to do. I believe that we should be thinking about "creating responses" rather than about "finding the answer." Besides depicting a more dynamic and participatory process, this phrase is a better reflection of what actually goes on in complex patient care situations.

Descriptive Research and Ethics Teaching

I turn now to some suggestions for curriculum reform derived from three descriptive research studies that address curriculum planning and development: the AACN study of the essentials of professional nursing education and two studies of ethical problems identified by nurses in hospitals and in the community. I discuss these studies because I believe they can contribute to the setting of priorities for objectives and content in curriculum.

The first study is one that I conducted at the University of Minnesota on ethical problems encountered by community health nurses. The sample was composed of staff nurses in community nursing agencies in the state of Minnesota who primarily delivered home care services. Major situations of ethical conflict were analyzed with an eye to determining how often a given situation was experienced by the respondents and how serious an ethical problem the situation posed. Among the situations identified by a majority of the respondents as severe ethical problems were inadequate care of client by self or family, lack of adequate information for decision making about treatment on the part of client or family, client incompetence to make or participate in major decisions, limited reimbursement for needed client care, disagreement with physician about treatment, misuse or abuse of medications by client or family, and questionable competency of other health professionals. Close to half of the respondents identified abuse of client rights, coercion of nursing staff by administration, questionable competency of nursing colleagues, and lack of administrative and collegial support for a working environment that enhanced quality client care as severe ethical problems. These findings point to areas that should not be neglected in nursing education.

Anne Davis (1981) conducted a survey of ethical dilemmas identified by respondents who were primarily hospital staff nurses. She found that the respondents had a good grasp of the concept of an ethical dilemma. The two most frequently occurring ethical dilemmas were prolonging life with heroic measures and unethical or incompetent activity on the part of colleagues. Davis (1979) also found that in conducting ethics rounds, nurses were aware of ethical dilemmas but were unable to articulate their ethical stance in a reasoned way. Her observations reinforce the mandate for change in nursing curricula.

The AACN baccalaureate data project (1987) included questions about ethical decision making. The 400 respondents were senior nursing students who were questioned before graduation and 6 to 12 months after graduation. Before graduation, 75 percent of the respondents viewed their nursing courses as sources for developing ethical decision-making abilities before graduation. Other sources were literature; courses in ethics in nursing school; courses in humanities, philosophy or ethics; courses in ethics outside of nursing; and ethics rounds in clinical practicum (17 percent). One year after graduation, 73 percent of the respondents perceived ethics content in nursing courses as sources for developing ethical decision-making abilities. Family influence was so perceived by 65 percent, group discussion of ethical dilemmas with colleagues and peers by 63 percent, religious influence by 63 percent, and courses in humanities, philosophy, logic, or ethics by 54 percent. Use of ethical frameworks or models was viewed as a source by only 23 percent.

The ethical dilemmas confronted by the 1984 senior nursing students 12 months after graduation included caring for patients with a poor prognosis or terminal illness, refusal of treatment by patients, initiating resuscitation, informed consent, and evaluation of patients' competence to make their own decisions. These dilemmas were experienced by at least half of the respondents. Allocation of scarce resources was a dilemma for only 12 percent of the respondents, in stark contrast with the findings from the community study.

CONCLUSIONS

Given the current state of ethics with respect to the nursing curriculum, present technological/political context, and the suggestions for objectives and content considered above, I would offer the following recommendations for the curriculum revolution in nursing.

1. The curriculum must be changed in such a way as to take into account both objectives and content in ethics and the settings within which nursing education occurs.
2. Since choices bearing on the development and use of technologies in nursing and health care are ethically and politically complex, we must study them carefully with an eye to determining how they and their consequences affect nursing curricula, caregivers, clients, and systems of care.
3. In order to act responsibly as faculty, we must not only use the knowledge and expertise we have in nursing but also ask colleagues in other fields (such as law, philosophy, political theory, and religious studies) to help us to develop more adequate responses to moral conflict in nursing for purposes of curriculum planning.

4. We must develop more collegially funded efforts in nursing scholarship that combine the expertise of nurses working in ethics with that of nurses studying clinical judgment; a good example is the work of Catherine Murphy and Marjory Gordon at Boston College.

Curriculum revolution in nursing education is a necessity, not a luxury. We can choose to put nursing intellect and energies into compassion, caring, and competence. To do otherwise is to fail in our duty to the clients of nursing education: future generations of nurses and the recipients of nursing care.

REFERENCES

American Association of Colleges of Nursing. (1987, November). Presentation given by Barbara K. Redman on Baccalaureate Data Project at Society for Health & Human Values Annual Meeting, Arlington, VA: Author.

American Nurses' Association. (1985). *Code for nurses with interpretive statements* (Publication No. G-56). Kansas City, MO: Author.

American Nurses' Association. (1980). *Nursing: A social policy statement* (Publication No. NP-63). Kansas City, MO: Author.

Aroskar, M. A. (1987). What happens to patient autonomy in high-tech care? *The American Nurse, 19*(4), 15.

Churchill, L. (1977). Ethical issues of a profession in transition. *American Journal of Nursing, 77*(5), 873–875.

Davis, A. J. (1979). Ethics rounds with intensive care nurses. *Nursing Clinics of Northern America, 14*(1), 45–55.

Davis, A. J. (1981). Ethical dilemmas in nursing: A survey. *Western Journal of Nursing Research, 3*(4), 397–407.

Fry, S. (1982). Ethical principles in nursing education and practice: A missing link in the unification issue. *Nursing & Health Care, 3*(7), 363–368.

Jameton, A. (1984). *Nursing practice: The ethical issues.* Englewood Cliffs, NJ: Prentice-Hall.

Noddings, N. (1984). *Caring: A feminine approach to ethics and moral education.* Berkeley: University of California Press.

Reiser, S. J., & Anbar, M. (Eds.). (1984). *The machine at the bedside.* New York: Cambridge University Press.

Schucking, E. L. (1985). Death at a New York hospital. *Law, Medicine Health-Care, 13*(6), 261–268.

Smith, R., & Brdlik, G. C. (1985). Medical devices: Where should learning begin? *Dean's Notes, 6,* 1.

Winner, L. (1986). *The whale and the reactor.* Chicago: University of Chicago Press.

9

Curriculum Revolution: A Theoretical and Philosophical Mandate for Change

Nancy Diekelmann

A curriculum revolution is only possible if true alternatives in nursing education are explored at both the curricular and the instructional level and if the process of nursing is reexamined. The model currently used in nursing education is the one that Tyler (1950) proposed several decades ago. Two alternative models also exist: phenomenological models and critical models. In this chapter, I will discuss these models, giving particular attention to one recently developed model, Curriculum as Dialogue and Meaning (Diekelmann, 1988b); which was formulated in an attempt to meet some of the challenges that remain to be addressed in nursing education. I will also consider some of the recommendations that have been made regarding the testing and implementation of these new curricular and instructional approaches, as well as the influence of our present accreditation process on their application. Perhaps a procedure should be established that would allow schools of nursing to petition for modification of the National League for Nursing's accreditation guidelines, so that they could explore new curricular alternatives without losing their accreditation or being put on warning. In any case, whether such a procedure is created or not, it is urgent that nursing educators and administrators find ways of working together to orchestrate a curriculum revolution.

The world of curriculum and curricular models abounds in feelings of frustration and futility. Today, however, another feeling presides. It is based on the recognition that the present curricular model is but one of the many models that can be used to organize nursing education. Disillusionment with the development and administration of nursing curricula is thus gradually being supplanted by excitement and new understanding as alternatives are developed.

The educational research of the curriculum reconceptualists, such as Apple (1979, 1982, 1986), Kliebard (1977, 1987), and Pinar (1975), makes it clear that there are two fundamental questions of curriculum that must be addressed by all models, new as well as old: How should the knowledge (subject matter) that nurses need to enter nursing practice safely be selected and sequenced? What is the role of experience in nursing education? It is also clear, however, that teachers, students, clinicians, nursing knowledge, and nursing practice all constantly change. Accordingly, the new curricular models approach schooling as a process in which the essential questions are constantly being asked and no answer is considered final. From this point of view, it is impossible to say that educators have "failed" when the curriculum is changed or modified every semester or every time a course is taught. If the curriculum is developed and organized according to a process model, it is continually scrutinized and adapted to meet the ever-changing nature of nursing practice.

Besides being practical, helpful, and efficient, curricular models should be flexible and allow for frequent change. The alternative models that have been proposed are less elaborate, appear to be less scientific, and require less attention to detail than the traditional model. Like creativity itself, they are not definite: they are guides rather than recipes. In what follows, I will begin with a brief discussion of the model in current use, focusing on some of its limitations, then proceed to a discussion of viable alternatives.

THE TYLER MODEL

The Tyler model (1950), which continues to be the standard for nursing education, provides the framework for NLN accreditation criteria. It was developed by Professor Ralph Tyler as the course syllabus for Education 360, a course taught at the University of Chicago in 1949. Over time, this document has come to pervade the thoughts of teachers to such an extent that it is difficult for us even to reexamine and reevaluate some of its central features, much less change it substantially or replace it.

The Tyler framework rests on four central questions:

1. What educational purposes should the school seek to attain?
2. What educational experiences can be provided that are likely to attain these purposes?
3. How can these educational experiences be effectively organized?
4. How can we determine whether these purposes are being attained?

Most commonly, these questions are considered to make up a four-step process comprising (1) statement of objectives, (2) selection of experiences, (3) organization of experiences, and (4) evaluation. The Tyler model is a linear means-ends process whose commonsense appeal conceals the taken-for-granted assumptions of an instrumentalist view of education.

Eisner (1985) provides a good description of the scientific and technical orientation of the Tyler framework:

> The scientific and technological orientation to curriculum is one that is *preoccupied* with the development of means to achieve prespecified ends. Those working from this orientation tend to view schooling as a complex system that can be analyzed into its constituent components. The problem for the educator or educational technologist is to bring the system under control so that the goals it seeks to attain can be achieved. (p. 44)

The Tyler model places high value on effectiveness, efficiency, certainty, and predictability, and it emphasizes individualism and competition. It assumes that knowledge consists of facts, generalizations, principles, laws, and theories, and that things can virtually always be explained by giving causal, functional, hypothetical, or deductive reasons. It also assumes that knowledge can be directly and easily translated into specific behaviors, and it emphasizes future outcomes while deemphasizing the "here and now." Furthermore, the model does not fully explain how teachers can decide which objectives to include in the curriculum and which to leave out; instead, it appeals to consensus and proposes the "common judgment of thoughtful men and women" as its criterion.

The Tyler model has numerous good points. For one, it requires teachers to expend a great deal of time and effort on deciding what will become subject matter for the nursing curriculum. Discussion of subject matter and the role of experience in nursing education are enhanced when teachers must specify both classroom and clinical objectives in great detail. Furthermore, the technical model of nursing education has been crucial in bringing nursing curricula out of hospitals and into almost every major university in the country within the space of 25 years. That was a major accomplishment on the part of those nurse educators of the 1960s who fought to legitimize nursing education and who were better grounded in the Tylerian model than most schools of education at the time. Some schools have developed exemplary nursing curricula based on the Tyler model and are expert at behavioral education.

Overall, the Tyler model has served us well to this point. Those schools in which this model works and is meaningful should not change simply for the sake of changing. But just as we must reconsider and revise our curricula periodically to take into account changes in students, faculty, clinical practice, and nursing knowledge, so must we also reconsider and, if necessary, revise the model on which the curricula are based. We must take advantage of the research in public education over the last 15 years and begin to consider alternative models.

The same model is used for accreditation as for instruction. It has many limitations, but here I will only mention one: the amount of time that the Tyler model forces nurse educators to spend on developing course and curriculum materials solely for the purpose of an accreditation visit. The model demands constant updating of these materials at a time when decisions about what to include and exclude from the curriculum are becoming more and more difficult to make. More than a few nurse educators are frustrated by having to prepare objectives solely because they are required, not because they are regularly used with students. For example, if at the end of the course a particular student receives a grade that seems unfair, the tool is adjusted on the basis of the objectives, and the final grade reflects what the teacher thinks is fair. Some instructors spend hours using clinical tools in an effort to be fair in grading students, when this time would be better spent reading and improving their own understanding of what they are teaching. The Tyler model has encouraged educators to focus on evaluation and data gathering and to use most of their time on clinical units in evaluating students. Likewise, faculty members spend most of their energies trying to organize the curriculum. It is time to explore some alternatives.

A QUEST FOR ALTERNATIVE ORIENTATIONS

The curricular literature of the 1970s reflected an interest in reconceptualizing the field of curriculum, exploring alternative paradigms or ideologies within which curriculum thought is embedded, and, most particularly, transcending behaviorism in curricular thought to embrace beingness and critical thought. Schools began to be viewed as places engaged in a search for situational meaning. During this time, the work of Eisner and Vallance (1974), Pinar and the reconceptualists (1975), Goodlad (1969), Apple (1979), and Freire (1970) manifested both a willingness to challenge the Tyler model and a desire to pursue alternative orientations. Educators must continue to explore these alternatives.

The Tyler Model as a Technical Model

The Tyler model is a technical model of education. One assumption of the technical model is that once students are given information in the classroom, they can then practice and apply it in the clinical area. Since reinforcement is important, it is considered desirable, by both students and teachers, to match a student who is studying diabetes with a diabetic patient, or a student studying problems of oxygenation with a hypoxic patient. Clinical checklists and course objectives are carefully coordinated with the aim of ensuring that students' learning is as strongly reinforced as students' clinical experience. The closer the match between theory and experience or between classroom and clinical instruction, the better and greater the learning.

A second assumption of the technical model is that all students should acquire some essential knowledge and skills. Implicit in this assumption is the notion that certain skills and knowledge should be identified by the faculty and practitioners as essential and taught to all students. Inevitably, some subject matter and skills continue to be taught even though students never encounter situations in which they can be used or practiced. There is, of course, considerable conflict among teachers regarding what knowledge and skills are essential. Sometimes this conflict raises questions of academic freedom. Schools that adhere strictly to the technical model prescribe subject matter and skills and require faculty to agree to teach the knowledge and skills identified as essential. The model assumes that faculty conflict should be resolved through compromise.

A third assumption of the technical model is that all students ought to have experience in every specialty area of nursing, or at least in as many as possible. This assumption may be operationalized as required community, operating room, or pediatric experience. Faculty, practitioners, and students alike embrace the notion that exposure to all specialty areas is essential if the student is to make appropriate employment and career choices after graduation.

Phenomenologic Models: Schools in Search of Meaning

In phenomenologic models of curriculum, the central concern is the communicative understanding of meanings given by people who live within the situation. These models (Greene, 1971; Huebner, 1975) acknowledge the possibility of multiple approaches to a phenomenon or problem. For example, it is possible to state objectives in a number of different ways, but in the final analysis it is the teacher who must interpret these printed statements and translate them into action. Instead of emphasizing the writing of objectives, phenomenologic models emphasize the processes of understanding that shape the world of the student and teacher. The written materials these models use can be identical to those used in the Tyler model; the crucial difference is that phenomenologic models of education emphasize the importance of experience and meaning.

The French existential phenomenologist Merleau-Ponty (1962) argued that a fuller understanding of any phenomenon requires a primary emphasis on how it is experienced:

> The whole universe of science is built upon the world as directly experienced, and if you want to subject science to rigorous study, we must begin by reawakening the basic experience of the world of which science is the second order experience. (p. 88)

The essence of the phenomenologic model is the attempt to come to some understanding of the world of Being, the lived world of people. The orientation is toward the here and now of the situation, and rules for the understanding of meaning are actively constructed by those who dwell within the situation.

The possibilities of the phenomenologic model for clinical education are great. In this model, clinicians develop the clinical courses in conjunction with faculty. One reason for the schism between education and practice may be that teachers feel they have to develop clinical objectives and then use them to evaluate students. Use of a phenomenologic model eliminates this emphasis on prediction and evaluation. Instead, it creates a focus on the lived experiences of clinicians and on introducing students into the clinical world. In this model, clinical nursing knowledge is an integral part of the curriculum, with practice informing the curriculum in much the same way that education has traditionally informed practice.

Teacher and student come together in the classroom, and the physical and social environment is transformed into a pedagogic situation. The essential process is not the transmission of information or the facilitation of learning, but the initiation and maintenance of dialogue. Knowing is not acquiring facts, but rather making meaning and giving meaning. To explain is to clarify common meanings and authenticate experiences. In this model, knowledge is not nomologic—that is, facts, laws, and theories—rather, it is situational meaning. This method is often used in case studies, and many teachers are at their best at those moments when they are engaging in dialogue with their students.

The phenomenologic model emphasizes the attempts of teachers-as-learners to understand the lived experiences of their students as well as their patients. To this end, expert clinicians are often brought into the classroom to lecture. Thus, teachers work with clinicians to establish exactly what the meaningful experiences—both clinical and classroom—are for students as they move from layperson to novice nurse and, for some, to graduate status. It is these life experiences within a lived situation that matter pedagogically. These experiences cannot be predicted or prescribed, but they can be demonstrated.

The role of the teacher is to seek ways of linking the contextual and conceptual worlds of students. Students need acontextual rules to help them enter new situations safely. Together, teacher and student seek to link the particular with the universal; the concrete, day-to-day, personal world of action with the world of ideas, values, and symbols, or, more generally, with systems of meaning. Not only are theory and practice integrated through action and reflection, but they also constitute part of a larger interpretive endeavor directed toward the recovery of meaning and the development of understanding. Clinical courses should build on each other as students develop their expertise. The necessary link between classroom (theory) and clinical experiences is thus deconstructed.

In the phenomenologic model, the private becomes more and more public. The main goal is to understand how and in what ways one becomes a nurse. Students have considerable private knowledge about what should be validated and made visible; thus, they are considered equal participants in the development of the curriculum. As their experiences are transformed into written documents for teachers, clinicians, and other students, these experiences may trigger valuable new insights into schooling. Teaching is a way of listening and responding, of hearing and heeding what is said. Listening is by no means a merely passive state: to be a listener presupposes that one not only is in a listening situation but also has actively taken up that situation as one's own. Teachers are the interpreters and historians who participate in a distinctive horizon of questions and experiences that throws open for students the future as possibility.

From this viewpoint, the curriculum is more than a set of objectives that serve as the parameters for the production of a nurse. Rather, it is the lived experiences of students, teachers, and clinicians as they work together in an attempt to understand how best to introduce students into the practice of nursing. The focus of the curriculum is the struggle to understand nursing knowledge and nursing practice. Caring, as an ontologic state, is fundamental to the curriculum.

Critical Models: Schools in Search of Critical Consciousness

Critical models also emphasize dialogue; where they differ from phenomenologic models is in their emphasis on a commitment to emancipation. Teachers who use these models seek to make visible to themselves and their students the power imbalances that occur in both our schools and our practice. They place high value on the critical processes of dialogue and debate, and they bring feminist and emancipatory approaches to the examination of issues confronting nursing students, both within the school and in the practice environment. Dialogue as a critical process is the foundation for this model.

Curriculum as Dialogue and Meaning

Curriculum as Dialogue and Meaning has points in common with both critical and phenomenologic models. It proposes an alternative way of conceptualizing nursing education that is based on a restructuring of the relationship between knowledge and skill acquisition. This restructuring profoundly affects how education, knowledge, experience, and expertise are defined and experienced in the nursing curriculum. In this model, the curriculum is a dialogue among teachers, practitioners, and students on what will constitute the knowledge in the nursing curriculum and what role experience will play in the curriculum. The curriculum is what it means to be a faculty-teacher-researcher, a practitioner-teacher, and a student nurse. The curriculum is both constituted and constituted by these people.

In Curriculum as Dialogue and Meaning, there is no higher court for discussions than the faculty, practitioners, and students involved. Dialogue is more than conversation; it is being-in-the-world with others through language and experience. In dialogue, it is assumed that decisions are only meaningful in the context in which faculty, students, and practitioners experience them. Thus, enlightened debate in which the issues and all the complexities involved, including those of power and control, are fully discussed does not necessitate a vote or consensus to become operational. To understand a "problem" from a new perspective is to understand what the problem means. The "solution," then, is achieved contextually, since all participants—teachers, practitioners, and students—will attend in their own way to the new meanings they have experienced.

Dialogue is a joint reflection on a phenomenon; it is a deepening of experience for all participants; it is talking, generating questions, and possibly interpreting. Dialogue involves the lived experiences of everyone and seeks shared understanding. Buber (1958) describes the "between," that is, the "seeing the between" or meeting to share a viewpoint as revealing and permitting understanding. According to Weber (1986), "it is through the seeing of that which is neither only *you* nor only *I*, but is rather *our* between that we learn about each other" (p. 68).

Curriculum as Dialogue and Meaning is a community of scholars, researchers, teachers, practitioners, and students who together think things through, glancing at the mirrors others hold up for them, discovering not only the other but also themselves. Dialogue is thus private and confidential, as well as social and public. It is oral discourse. Accordingly, in this model the definition of curriculum as a set of beliefs that provide a framework that guides selecting and sequencing of courses in a school is replaced by a process (dialogue) that acknowledges all as participants in the curriculum and as human beings of importance—people who understand education, research, and nursing. Dialogue is respectful, open, and responsible, and it implies a willingness to learn.

The "problems" of the curriculum are "solved" through open questioning in dialogue. Heidegger (1962) argues that "the very act of posing a question is disclosure, for to question is to sketch in advance the context of meaning in which a particular inquiry will move." The answering in turn invites more questioning, thereby also guiding the dialogue. The dialogue is thus shaped by all, becoming, for the moment, "their shared abode" (Weber, 1986, p. 68).

Sometimes dialogue permits faculty, practitioners, and students to experience the "meaningful silence" of listening and thinking, in which they may participate more through gestures than through speech. Dialogue is experiencing moments of judgment and emotional reactions. These reactions may be unspoken: one party may simply be thinking, "How interesting," or "I know how she feels, that happened to me too," or perhaps "How different from my own experience this is." Still, dialogue must always affect everyone involved, or it is not dialogue. It continues long after the participants have departed. It is often experienced in the form of recollection or reflection. "I wish I had asked . . . ," or "I'd like to know. . . ." According to Weber (1986), "One dialogue echoes thoughts of another and through persons, ideas are exchanged, challenged, and tested" (p. 69).

COMPARISON OF THE TECHNICAL MODEL WITH THE CURRICULUM AS DIALOGUE AND MEANING

In Curriculum as Dialogue and Meaning, knowledge is instrumental, practical, and critical. Experience is defined as the turning around of preconceived notions, or the refining and elaborating of previously held beliefs, skills, and expertise (Heidegger, 1962). Expertise is the ability to theorize using knowledge that is instrumental, practical, and critical.

As noted earlier, the technical model makes two important assumptions: that it is necessary to identify essential knowledge and skills for the curriculum, and that it is desirable to reinforce and match theory with clinical experiences. In Curriculum as Dialogue and Meaning, the curriculum is reconceptualized as containing two kinds of knowledge: one kind instrumental and theoretical and the other practical and dependent on experience—in other words, "knowing that" and "knowing how." "Knowing that" knowledge is instrumental and is that part of the curriculum taught in the classroom by teachers who are expert in theoretical knowledge. "Knowing how" knowledge is practical: It is acquired through the clinical experience of nursing and is found in the practitioners or clinical faculty. This knowledge is not, however, taught by the practitioners or the clinical faculty, because clinical knowledge cannot be taught; it can only be demonstrated. It is personal, and it can only be acquired through experience. Thus, expertise in nursing education is the use of "knowing that" knowledge to aid the development of "knowing how" knowledge in the context of nursing practice. In Curriculum as Dialogue and Meaning, the objective of clinical learning is the development of the clinical expertise of the student. This expertise is defined as the ability to make clinical decisions that take context into account. It involves clinical decision making, but in a sense that is fundamentally different from that typically captured by descriptions of the nursing process.

The objective of developing clinical expertise in students does not depend on a corresponding relationship between classroom and clinical instruction. The clinical courses can be conceptualized in relation to the development of expertise, while the classroom courses can be conceptualized in terms of the selection and sequencing of nursing knowledge. Since learning is not defined as the transfer or application of information, it is not mandatory that the student demonstrate to the teacher the transfer of a skill from one setting to another or that information in the classroom be matched with phenomena in the clinical area. For example, it is not required that students apply information in their care plans to show teachers that they can do so accurately. Thus, the elaborate coordination of classroom and clinical teaching, based on assumptions of reinforcement and a corresponding relationship between theory and practice, is not necessary.

This is not to say, however, that the selection and sequencing of subject matter for the curriculum is eliminated, for it is important that faculty, practitioners, and students spend time determining how classroom content should be presented. What is desired is a wedding of the acontextual rules of the specialty areas with the emerging clinical decision-making skills. The relationship between theory and practice, or theoretical knowledge and practical knowledge, is transactional rather than applicational. The practice area is the place where students enter into dialogue with the theories they learn in the classroom. It is through practice that theories are refined, elaborated, and challenged. Practice is theory-generating, and in this sense, as Heidegger's notions (1962) of practical knowledge preceding theoretical knowledge suggest, theoretical concerns are derivative.

Classroom and clinical learning intersect at the epistomologic level. According to the research done on clinical decision making (Benner, 1984), student nurses use rule-governed behavior to enter new nursing situations safely. The challenge for the theoretical faculty who teach in the classroom is to identify the knowledge students need for safe entry into nursing situations through the study of nursing and related fields. Today, the rules of nursing are more deeply entrenched in our textbooks and literature than ever, and the essential task for classroom teachers is to determine, through research and the generation of nursing knowledge, what rules and knowledge are actually necessary. The challenge for the clinical faculty, on the other hand, is to attempt, through research, to understand how students acquire clinical decision-making skills in nursing, as well as how they use experience to acquire nursing expertise.

The curriculum also contains what is known as critical knowledge, which is concerned with making overt and conscious the issues of power and control that affect the curriculum at all levels. This knowledge seeks to provide faculty, students, and clinicians with the greatest amount of freedom through dialogue while identifying the issues of power and control that dominate and limit such freedom within the context of the curriculum. However, the issues of power and control are never limited to the curriculum alone. Thus, the notion of "essential knowledge" is one in which all faculty, practitioners, and students have an equal interest.

Curriculum as Dialogue and Meaning contests the notion that there can be "consensual validation" of "essential knowledge." Research in education (Greene, 1971; Kliebard, 1977, 1987) showed long ago that faculty consensus on issues of subject matter tends to identify knowledge that is either obvious or trivial. For example, who would argue that nursing students do not need to know how to give an intramuscular injection safely? Consensus on this point would be easy to obtain, but it would be little more than common sense.

Dialogue raises the discussion to another level. More sophisticated questions are asked. For example, how proficient in critical care skills should baccalaureate and associate degree students be? Should they be required to develop their skill in intravenous therapy? Should mock code situations be required or optional for students? In this kind of a discussion, everyone's interest is apparent. Faculty who are generating knowledge about advanced nursing practice are concerned that students have the skills they will need to use the knowledge being generated; practitioners desire that students have the skills they need to care for the patients they are assigned; and students want the skills they need to care for patients safely both while they are in school and after they have graduated. Dialogue among faculty, practitioners, and students on what knowledge and skills are to be taught allows freer determination of classroom knowledge. Similar dialogue occurs in the identification of clinical learning experiences.

In Curriculum as Dialogue and Meaning, students need not have at least one experience in each specialty area, nor are particular specialty areas or experiences mandatory. A school may decide to impose certain requirements, after dialogue with faculty, practitioners, and students, but the rationale would not be—as it is today—that students would thereby be better prepared to select the area in which they are most skilled and would most like to practice after graduation. These choices are best left to the student's discretion.

The rationale for specifying clinical experience rests not on the job needs of the specialty but rather on the needs of the patient populations being served. Thus, it is possible to learn about caring for the chronically ill by caring for either children or adults. This is not to imply that these two groups do not have very different needs. However, if the objective of clinical instruction is to help students learn the appropriate rule-governed behavior as a part of acquiring the nursing expertise necessary to care for someone with a chronic illness, the patient population is but one variable. The provision of experiences for novice nurses that lead them from rule-governed behavior to the development of a sense of generalizable attributes and aspects is possible in any nursing specialty.

Allowing students to control the rate at which they change nursing specialty areas and nursing units is supported by research in which student nurses reported that constantly learning new units and nursing specialties interfered with their ability to enter and experience the nursing culture (Diekelmann, 1988a). The students reported understanding, and in some instances accepting, the "cold reception" they received as being legitimate, since they felt that they often did not know what they were doing and had many questions that staff had to answer.

In Curriculum as Dialogue and Meaning, attention is paid to the issues of socialization as well as to the learning of the necessary clinical judgment skills. This model is based on the development of new collaborative relationships between teachers and practitioners that would allow all hospitals to be laboratories for students learning nursing, and that would allow nurses to experience as a part of schooling a caring environment in which they are valued by all nurses as a rich resource for the profession. New titles and creative use of hospital and teaching positions can make new levels of collaboration possible. For example, professor-clinicians who are doctorally prepared but hospital-based could as part of their clinical assignment contribute to the learning of clinical students at all levels. Placing master's students, two senior students, two junior students, and four sophomore students, all with different objectives, on a single unit could give students the opportunity to experience the nursing culture in new ways as they develop their skills and expertise in nursing. Staff nurses could be involved in clinical instruction in ways that are not dependent on classroom activities. Students could choose either to stay on a unit or in an agency for more than one semester or to specialize, which would enable them to experience the nursing culture over time.

Allowing students the option of selecting clinical experiences at the baccalaureate level is also supported by much of the research done on clinical decision making. Benner (1984) has documented that it is through developing a sense of attributes and aspects that expertise is developed in novices. To develop these aspects and attributes in a more general sense, the students must have enough similar experiences to make the appropriate judgments. For example, to learn when to make the clinical judgment of whether a particular blood pressure is meaningfully low or whether a patient is cyanotic, the student must have enough experiences in which the opportunity to make these qualitatively graded decisions is available. One way of maximizing this kind of decision-making experience is to give students the chance to control patient populations.

Curriculum as Dialogue and Meaning reconceptualizes the curriculum and the assumptions regarding knowledge, experience, and expertise implicit in it. There are other important assumptions regarding temporality, being, and language that have not been explicated but that also underlie the model.

INSTRUCTIONAL ALTERNATIVES

Empowering

One instructional alternative worth considering is a pedagogy that is *empowering*. Such an approach would have as a major concern the development of students' powers of inquiry, self-knowledge, and ability to make and remake knowledge and culture. Teachers have always been attentive to the intellectual development of students, but an empowering pedagogy would place more emphasis on this process than on content (Shor, 1980). The goal would be to avoid reproducing curricula that are so full of information that there is little time to talk to students and few activities for students to think critically in.

It will not be easy to find ways to have dialogue with students in today's crowded curriculum; lectures do not easily lend themselves to anything besides simple transmission of information. Nevertheless, there are strategies that can be used. Language and thinking are intimately linked. The use of a variety of writing experiences across the curriculum might help students to develop their critical skills. Such experiences include critiquing syllabi, not for what they include but for what they exclude. Helping students understand the critical processes clinicians and teachers bring to nursing will help them to understand the nature of critical thinking in nursing practice. It is timely to explore ways of thinking about and organizing care other than in care plans, which are poor reflections of the kind of critical processes used in practice.

An increasingly important issue in nursing is the ethical quagmires that nurses are facing more and more often in practice. Dialogue with clinicians can only enhance the critical abilities of students as they enter nursing practice.

Reconciliation

A second alternative to consider is *reconciliation* between students and teachers to reduce hostility and to foster solidarity instead of alienation. Research based on interviews of student nurses shows that students continue to be extremely fearful (Diekelmann, 1988a). This is not a new observation; indeed, the power and control teachers wield in nursing has been a recurring theme throughout the history of nursing education. Though teachers take considerable pains to try to create supportive environments in which students can learn and grow while protecting patients and providing optimum care, novice students are still extremely fearful of teachers. Something is wrong, and teachers need to enter into dialogue with their students to find out what that might be. Talking with students about their lived experiences and their reactions to the curriculum may help create new relationships with them (Diekelmann, 1988a).

In a number of studies, students reported that they did not trust faculty. They talked about "playing the game" and "psyching out the teacher." One student said, "What is playing the game? It's knowing what to do and what not to do, what counts and what doesn't, who to talk to and about what—that's what it is." Teachers need to explore why students are so suspicious. Certainly this will be difficult with students who have constantly been talked at and told what to do and not to do throughout their educational careers. Lack of motivation and apathy—or, in Shor's (1986) phrase, performance strikes—on the part of those students should not be surprising. Nonetheless, if teachers put their energies into understanding the student experience, it may prove possible to transform their relationships with them. Teachers might then be better able to engage students in the recreation of the nursing curriculum.

Situated Study

A third alternative is *situated study*, a pedagogy in which the study of one exercise merges into another. It is flexible and fluid and allows teachers to abandon the syllabus or the topic to be discussed when the students become engaged in a topic that is of interest to them.

Certainly teachers are under restrictions that may present them from being this flexible, but there are times when they might seek to engage students. In the Diekelmann (1988a) study, a student talks about her frustration in negotiating a paper topic. She said, "Those primary courses are really exciting to me because I didn't have any community health in my nursing program before. Like I was saying before, any *new* stuff is really exciting. I love it really a lot. But repetition is hard. I don't think I'm so smart that I can't learn more, but it's just that sometimes you just sit there and like *you've heard it and you remember it*. . . ."

This student nurse reminds me of a student on strike—a serious strike in which she is bored and unchallenged and finds the experience "demeaning." Shor (1986) describes this kind of student strike well:

> Students will resist any process that disempowers them. Unequal, disabling education is symbolic violence against them, which they answer with their own skills of resistance—silence, disruption, nonperformance, cheating, lateness, absence, vandalism, etc. Very familiar school routines produce this alienation: teacher-talk, passive instruction in preset materials, punitive testing, . . . denial of themes and other subjects important to them, the exclusion of student coparticipation in curriculum design and governance. . . .

The nurse quoted earlier provides a concrete example of why students strike. "For example," she recalled,

> I, we had to talk, give a presentation on something within the nursing field or the health medical field, and I talked about the homeless, and in my critique my teacher couldn't understand what they had to do with the health field and just went on to say that she really didn't understand what my point was of speaking on the homeless. And I had to proceed to tell her that it was an evergrowing problem, especially now when people, if people don't have

> insurance, don't have access to the medical services, then people are sicker, people aren't seeking out the care they need. And she just, I don't know, we kind of went around and around about why I thought that was important and why I thought that had to do with something in the medical field. I don't know, I had a hard time with her. As a person, I got along with her.

It is ironic that this student provides an example that reflects the very solution to transforming education. According to Shor (1986),

> The vast alienation of students from school and society can drown any plan that does not empower them to transform reality, to study their culture critically and to remake it. Situated study can reverse these conditions. Any curriculum opaqueing reality instead of illuminating it, against student equality and aspirations, will sink in an ocean of rejection. (pp. 182–183)

Many students are not used to directing their own study, so it will be difficult for them initially. Perhaps giving teachers the permission to abandon the topic to be discussed or the assignment that is required by all to engage in a meaningful topic is a good place to begin. In this way intuition, imagination, and experimentation can become valued methods of learning. Knowledge is not a fixed thing to be swallowed whole: it is invented in each class. The excitement of learning is the "making of meaning."

Teacher Work

Finally, it is necessary to take a brief look at teacher work. If teacher work is a form of intellectual labor, then how can the fundamental nature of the conditions under which we work be redefined and changed? Can we imagine a role for the teacher not as information giver or facilitator of learning but rather as learner and intellectual? Through dialogue, we could begin to do away with the widespread separation of the conceptualization of the curriculum, the planning, and the design from the nature of teacher work itself. A good first step would be to reject those conceptual frameworks that do not seem meaningful to either teachers or students.

Through dialogue, all participants in the educational process struggle to create the structural and emotional environment that is necessary for the faculty to practice, write, research, and work with each other. Faculty members are in need of empowerment as well, and the empowering stories they share with each other should speak not only of how to promote achievement or advance students along a career ladder, but also how to help students read the world of nursing critically so that they can change it through struggle and community.

NURSING CURRICULAR AND INSTRUCTIONAL MODELS: ACCREDITATION AND INNOVATION

Given nursing education's close historical ties to the larger world of education, it is curious that there has not been more experimentation with these alternative curricular models. A study I recently conducted with Professors Chris Tanner and David Allen (1988) revealed that the Tyler model was used to the exclusion of other models in determining accreditation criteria. Thus, to explore and implement these new models on the curricular level is to fail to meet the accreditation criteria spelled out for the curriculum. Although the criteria were not intended to make innovation and research on alternative curricular models impossible, their effect is restrictive nonetheless.

Lack of funding for educational research has also made large nursing curriculum research programs impossible. Given that declining enrollments have created a nursing shortage and students who enter nursing curricula are also consumers of educational programs, it seems obvious that research on alternatives in nursing education is urgently needed. Many innovative programs have already been initiated. In some, educators are using only a few innovative approaches; in others, they are fighting for full accreditation for their innovative curricula. What is needed is dialogue and increased interest in exploring and researching these new approaches in nursing. The entry into practice, whether or not it will ever be formally passed, has made many nurses realize that they should consider getting baccalaureate degrees. These students are coming back to nursing schools, and curricula must be developed to meet their needs; if this is not done, they will spread the word that nothing has really changed in nursing education. All the effort that has been put into increasing the educational levels of nurses will have been wasted. Research and exploration of curricular models for RN students are desperately needed. One such alternative model is the RN-to-MS program.

It is still believed in many circles that educational research is not nursing research. Assistant professors are encouraged to develop clinical nursing research programs so that they can meet tenure criteria.

Often, nurses obtain their PhD in education, but find that when they return to schools of nursing, they are forced to develop research programs in nursing rather than in nursing education in order to obtain funding. The widespread view of educational research as nonscholarly and dominated by evaluation studies must be reevaluated. The Society for Research in Nursing Education needs members and support in order to raise the visibility of scholarly research in nursing education and to increase pressure to restore funding for nursing education.

It may be that teachers are discouraged because they seem to be reinventing the wheel when they try to revise curricula. They have been sold many "true alternatives" that were really nothing more than variations on the Tyler model. As a result they have begun to ask themselves whether any real alternatives exist. Many of us remember when instructional technology was going to revolutionalize education. Today, however, the era of the "talking heads" has come and gone, and educators are faced with yet another curriculum revolution. What is different about this revolution is that the questions are the same, but there is no attempt to dictate the outcome. The selection and sequencing of subject matter and the role of experience in education are basic questions; what is different now is that the curriculum is considered to be a process that often brings teachers, students, and clinicians together to talk about these questions. The curriculum should change often, because students, teachers, and clinical practices change, as does nursing knowledge itself. Thus, the struggle to develop a set of criteria that will guide the process is replaced with a series of questions that teachers will always struggle with and that will be answered differently in different contexts.

Teachers must acknowledge their lived experiences with the technical model and try to evaluate, through dialogue, just how fruitful it has been. For example, would educators labor endlessly over objectives if they were not required? Would they spend as much time discussing the framework of the curriculum in curriculum meetings if that were not a part of accreditation? Is there any evidence that well-written and tightly constructed curricula produce excellence in schools of nursing? What actually contributes to excellence in schools of nursing? Is it time for educators to enter into dialogue about the meaningful and meaningless activities they engage in as teachers? Would the one hour a day spent doing clinical evaluations be better spent talking with students? Research on the accreditation process in nursing is desperately needed. Discussion of the assets and limitations of the technical model will help teachers begin to explore other possibilities while grounding them in nursing history. Perhaps pilot projects similar to the open curriculum projects initiated during the 1970's should be started across the country to encourage exploration of alternative curricular models and alternative accreditation criteria. (Notter & Robey, 1979).

TRANSCENDING BEHAVIORISM AND INSTRUMENTALISM IN CURRICULUM ORIENTATION

Once again, it is absolutely essential that educators have dialogue about alternatives in nursing curricula, if they are to take advantage of the new possibilities that are rising in the current curriculum revolution. They must also have dialogue regarding changes in the accreditation process. Perhaps pilot schools across the country could petition for suspension of the NLN accreditation criteria and replacement of these criteria with criteria and a process that would allow the schools to experiment with new curricular models without being put on warning. Most of all, educators must continue to talk with colleagues who fought diligently to bring the technical model into nursing and into accreditation to ensure that errors are not made. These collegial voices will help others to understand what it means to make fundamental changes in nursing education. Educators should learn from Professor Tyler, whose "new" model for the curriculum now enslaves us, and be wary of all new models, including such alternatives as Curriculum as Dialogue and Meaning. In conclusion, it is time for us as educators to revisit our curricular and instructional models and struggle with the fundamental question of how best to school men and women into nursing practice.

REFERENCES

Apple, M. (1979). *Ideology and curriculum.* London: Routledge & Kegan Paul.

Apple, M. (Ed.). (1982). *Cultural and economic reproduction in education.* London: Routledge & Kegan Paul.

Apple, M. (1986). *Teachers and texts.* London: Routledge & Kegan Paul.

Benner, P. (1984). *From novice to expert: Excellence and power in clinical nursing practice.* Menlo Park, CA: Addison-Wesley.

Buber, M. (1958). *I and thou.* New York: Scribners.

Diekelmann, N. (1988a). *From layperson to novice nurse: The lived-experiences of nursing students.* Unpublished manuscript, School of Nursing, University of Wisconsin, Madison.

Diekelmann, N. (1988b). *The curriculum as dialogue and meaning.* Unpublished manuscript, School of Nursing, University of Wisconsin, Madison.

Eisner, E. (1985). *The educational imagination: On design and evaluation of school programs.* New York: Macmillan.

Eisner, E., & Vallance E. (1974). *Conflicting conceptions of curriculum.* Berkeley, CA: McCutchan.

Freire, P. (1970). *Pedagogy of the oppressed.* New York: Herder and Herder.

Goodlad, J. (1969). Curriculum: State of the field. *Review of Educational Research, 39,* 367–88.

Greene, M. (1971). Curriculum and consciousness. *Teachers College Record, 73*(2), 253–69.

Heidegger, M. (1962). *Being and time.* (J. Macquarrie & E. Robinson, Trans.). New York: Harper & Row.

Huebner, D. (1975). The tasks of the curricular theorist. In W. Pinar (Ed.), *Curriculum theorizing—The reconceptualists.* Berkeley, CA: McCutchan.

Kliebard, H. (1977). The Tyler rationale. In W. Pinar (Ed.), *Curriculum and evaluation,* (pp. 56–67). Berkeley, CA: McCutchan.

Kliebard, H. (1987). *The struggle for the American curriculum, 1893–58.* London: Routledge & Kegan Paul.

Merleau-Ponty, M. (1962). *The phenomenology of perception.* Atlantic Highlands, NJ: The Humanities Press.

Notter, L., & Robey, M. (1979). *The open curriculum in nursing education* (Publication No. 19-1799). New York: National League for Nursing.

Pinar, W. (Ed.). (1975). *Curriculum theorizing: The reconceptualists.* Berkeley, CA: McCutchan.

Shor, I. (1980). *Critical teaching and everyday life.* Chicago: The University of Chicago Press.

Shor, I. (1986). *Culture wars: Schools and society in the conservative restoration, 1969–1984.* London: Routledge & Kegan Paul.

Tanner, C., Diekelmann, N., & Allen, D. (1988). *The National League for Nursing criteria for appraisal of baccalaureate programs: A critical hermeneutical analysis.* New York: National League for Nursing.

Tyler, R. (1950). *Basic principles of curriculum and instruction.* Chicago: The University of Chicago Press.

Weber, S. (1986). The nature of interviewing. *Phenomenology + Pedagogy, 4*(2), 65–70.

10

Implications of Clinical Judgment Research for Teaching

Sheila A. Corcoran and Christine Tanner

Most of the participants at this conference would agree that the development of competence in clinical judgment is as essential to the goal of nursing education as it is to the practice of safe and effective nursing care. Despite this agreement, there has been very little research related to teaching clinical judgment in nursing. In the 20 years from 1966 to 1986, approximately 50 studies were reported in the literature (Tanner, 1987). This paper will briefly examine the research literature to derive potential strategies for teaching clinical reasoning. Five of these strategies will be described in some detail. The paper will conclude by examining the implications of clinical judgment research for curriculum planning.

ASSUMPTIONS

Several assumptions support this paper. The first is that clinical judgment and decision making require both knowledge and decision-making skills. As Simon (1979) pointed out, there is no expertise without extensive and accessible knowledge. Yet knowledge alone is not enough. Processes for operating on that knowledge to solve problems and to answer questions are also needed.

The second assumption is that clinical reasoning can be taught.

There is little research evidence to support this assumption, but making it seems essential to our well-being as educators.

The third assumption is that while specific tasks may require particular thinking skills and strategies, there are general skills for processing knowledge to solve problems and answer questions. Frederiksen (1984) pointed out that instruction concerned with unknown ill-structured problems of the future requires generality; basic skills with wide applicability as well as general processes, such as use of heuristics and strategies, should be taught.

The final assumption, which is related to the second one, is that humans have the capability to transfer skills and knowledge from specific situations to analagous but not identical situations.

An issue related to these assumptions is the paradox of expertise. While we would like to know how experts think and to teach novices to think accordingly, experts are usually unable to describe how they perform their tasks. They reach a level of "automaticity" in which they perform tasks without thinking about it; their knowledge is tact knowledge, unavailable to consciousness (Johnson, 1983). Despite this paradox, researchers have found ways to reveal and infer thinking processes. Critics of these methods, however, caution that the resulting theories may be based on naivete, since the expert is least able to reproduce his or her thought processes.

SUMMARY OF RESEARCH ON TEACHING CLINICAL JUDGMENT

The research related to teaching clinical judgment conducted over the last 20 years falls into four major categories: (1) strategies for teaching clinical judgment; (2) measures of clinical judgment performance; (3) factors associated with performance in clinical judgment; and (4) processes of judgment (Tanner, 1987).

In the five studies investigating approaches to teaching clinical judgment (Aspinall, 1979; deTornyay, 1968a; Mitchell & Atwood, 1975; Tanner, 1982), no approach resulted in both meaningful and statistically significant improvement in clinical judgment performance. It should be noted that there has been no study of the usefulness of our most firmly rooted instructional approach—the written nursing care plan.

To date, several studies have examined reliability and validity of written simulations as measures of clinical judgment performance (deTornyay, 1968b; Dincher, & Stidger, 1976; Farrand, Holzemer, &

Schleutermann, 1982; McIntyre, McDonald, Bailey, & Claus, 1972; McLaughlin, Carr, & Deluchi, 1981). While these measures have satisfactory reliability, their relationship to performance in actual practice remains to be established. Holzemer (1986), a well-known investigator in the field of problem-solving simulations, concluded that they lack sufficient validity to place confidence in them as the only method of evaluation.

In the search for factors associated with performance in clinical judgment, investigators have examined test scores on critical thinking appraisal, personality type, and years of education and experience, among other variables (Davis, 1972; Davis, 1974; del Bueno, 1983; Frederickson & Mayer, 1977; Gordon, 1980; Koehne-Kaplan & Tilden, 1976; Verhonick, Nichols, Glor, & McCarthy, 1968). In several studies, a positive correlation between years of education and measures on a problem-solving simulation was demonstrated (Davis, 1972; Davis, 1974; del Bueno, 1983; Verhonick et al., 1968). A curvilinear relationship between years of experience and performance has also been shown in at least two studies, with nurses with up to four years and more than six to ten years showing poorer performance against those with years of experience in the middle range. It may be that the paradox of expertise shows up in these studies.

In the final category, numerous studies have been conducted to explore the processes of clinical judgment (Corcoran, 1986a; Corcoran, 1986b; Gordon, 1980; Grier, 1976; Pyles & Stern, 1983; Tanner, Padrick, Westfall, & Putzier, 1987; Westfall, Tanner, Putzier, & Padrick, 1986). These studies are aimed at three types of questions: (1) how do expert nurses select relevant information from the vast amount of clinical data which is available to a particular situation; (2) how do nurses infer from this information the patient's health status or responses to changing health status; and (3) how do nurses determine what interventions are appropriate? Researchers investigating these questions are apparently motivated by the notion that a better understanding of expert performance in the processes of clinical judgment will enable nurses to teach these processes to students.

Examples of studies addressing these questions were presented in the plenary session by Tanner. Although the results from these studies are far from conclusive, some tentative conclusions which may be useful for design of instruction strategies are offered: (1) Clinicians probably use both analytic and intuitive processes. In analytic processes, the situation is broken down into component elements; a judgment is made by a rational combination of these elements. In intuitive processes, the situation is taken as a whole. The contrast between these two processes is exemplified by a diagnostic task; using analysis, the clinician would examine each cue, weigh diagnostic hypotheses against each cue, then select the hypothesis with the highest probability of being correct, given the cues which are present. Using intuition, the clinician would attain a grasp of the whole situation, recognize those aspects of it which are salient or recognize a pattern as being similar or dissimilar to known patterns. (2) Performance in clinical judgment is context-dependent and dependent on the nature of the patient situation, as well as on the clinician's past experience with similar situations. The extent to which skills and processes of clinical judgment learned through familiar situations transfer to unfamiliar situations is not known. (3) There is some evidence that experts use strategies of heuristics in their decision making. Examples include the generation of diagnostic hypotheses early in the encounter, and the use of these hypotheses to guide subsequent acquisition of additional clinical data. The extent to which these heuristics can be taught to novices is not known, nor is it known what their effect would be if they were taught. Would they indeed be helpful to the novice in his or her decision making?

Although knowledge of the cognitive processes involved in clinical decision making is far from complete, and information on instructional methods and their value is even more incomplete, it seems that we cannot ignore the need to teach this content. We must proceed on the basis of the knowledge we have available to us to develop a repertoire of approaches for teaching clinical reasoning.

SELECTED TEACHING STRATEGIES

In a recent article on the implications of cognitive theory for instruction in problem solving, Frederiksen (1984) emphasized three aspects of problem solving: problem representation, problem-solving procedures, and pattern recognition. He pointed out that an accurate and complete problem representation provides a decision maker with a mental scheme containing factual and procedural knowledge for solving a particular kind of problem. The second aspect, problem-solving procedures, gives a decision maker a repertoire of strategies, heuristics, and plans for dealing with a particular situation. The third aspect, pattern recognition, provides a way of "chunking" information in order to deal with the limitations of short-term memory.

This section will describe several teaching strategies which promote the development of these three aspects of problem solving, beginning with two related to developing problem representations: analogies and decision analysis. After each strategy is described, it will be illustrated in practice, identified by its theoretical basis, and provided empirical support, if any.

Developing Problem Representations

Analogies. Analogies can be used for problem representation to simplify the mental image of a task, or to view a situation from another perspective. Recall analogies are often used in patient education to help persons develop simple mental images of their physical status. For example, consider the analogy frequently used to represent the heart and circulatory system as a closed system of circulating fluids, with the heart serving as a pump.

The Synectic Model of teaching is one instructional approach which incorporates analogies. It has five phases: (1) describe the present situation or problem; (2) present and describe an analogy for the situation; (3) describe the similarities between the analogy and the situation; (4) describe the differences between the analogy and the situation; and (5) re-explore the original situation on its own terms (Joyce & Weil, 1986).

The following example illustrates the Synectic Model and the use of an analogy to help nursing students develop a simple but powerful mental representation. A teacher was trying to help undergraduate nursing students gain a perspective of patients as persons, that is, whole human beings. The students were having difficulty. They repeatedly referred to human beings as a combination of biological, psychological, social, and spiritual parts. To counter this, in the next class the teacher used an analogy as an instructional strategy to represent holism. The teacher came with several props. First the teacher described the situation of having difficulty grasping the concept of holism. Then the teacher set out jars of flour, water, sugar, butter, eggs, and baking powder on the table. The teacher asked, "What do I have here?" The students listed the ingredients. Then the teacher took all the ingredients out of the jars, put them into a bowl, mixed them together and asked, "What do I have now?" The students indicated a mixture of the ingredients. The next question was, "Can I retrieve any of the individual ingredients?" to which the answer was "No." Next the teacher said, "Imagine that I have put these mixed ingredients into a pan and placed them in an oven at 350 degrees for one hour. Here is what I have," as she revealed a cake. Then the teacher asked the students to describe the analogy. The students stated: "We ended up with something very different from the ingredients with which we began, a cake"; "The separate ingredients to make the cake are not visible"; "The ingredients cannot be pulled out"; and "A transformation occurred in the ingredients as they were mixed and heated." Next the students were asked to describe the similarities between the cake and a whole person. The students repeated the statements about the inability to distinguish or extract the parts, whether of a cake or a person. They talked about a cake being different from and greater than the sum of the ingredients, just as persons are different from and greater than the sum of their parts. The students also indicated that one could examine the parts, for example, the quality of the flour or the quality of a person's heart; and the quality of the parts could influence the quality of the whole, but did not describe the whole. Next, the students discussed the differences between a cake and a person. Then they reexamined their problem with the concept of holism.

The Synectic Model was developed by William Gordon (1970) to increase problem-solving capability, creative expression, and insight. Metaphoric activity is the process used. Metaphors, in the form of analogies, establish likeness by comparing one object or idea with another object or idea, and by using one in place of the other. Through these substitutions the creative process occurs, connecting the familiar with the unfamiliar or creating a new idea from familiar ideas.

There are few cognitive processes that have undergone more intensive investigation in the past decade than those underlying analogical reasoning (Holyoak, 1984; Sternberg, 1983). In a recent study, Alexander, White, Haensley, and Crimmins-Jeanes (1987) demonstrated that analogy training can be effectively provided in the classroom with both young and older students. In addition, they found that the effects of training are maintained for at least a six-week period and are transferred to performance on analogy tasks different from those directly trained.

Decision Analysis. Decision analysis, another instructional strategy for promoting problem representation, provides a structure for depicting decision tasks. It is useful for helping learners develop a representation of alternative actions, possible chance events, possible outcomes, and values.

There are four steps to decision analysis: (1) structure a decision flow diagram composed of alternatives, chance events, and possible outcomes; (2) assign values to each set of possible outcomes; (3) assign probabilities to chance events; (4) calculate expected values; and (5) choose the alternative with the highest expected value (Corcoran, 1986b).

The first step provides the structure to represent a problem. In steps 2 through 5, decision analysis also provides a process for combining information to arrive at a best decision. Therefore, in addition to problem representation, decision analysis can be used as a teaching strategy to help develop problem-solving procedures, the second aspect of problem solving to be addressed later.

Only the first two steps of decision analysis will be illustrated here in a situation in which a group of hospice nurses wanted to simply represent the problem of titrating analgesic dosage to control a patient's pain. They reviewed related literature and found it inconclusive, with some articles and research studies recommending a high dosage initially and a downward titration and others recommending a low dosage and an upward titration. The nurses decided to use decision analysis to structure the problem in a hypothetical situation and to help them identify the information they needed to know and use.

In step one, the nurses developed the decision flow diagram shown in Figure 1. It consisted of two alternatives: starting with a high dosage of oral morphine solution and titrating downward or starting with a low dosage and titrating upward. The two chance events (states of nature over which the decision maker has no control) for each alternative were the occurrences of analgesic effects and of physiologic side effects. The set of outcomes of major concern included the rapidity of pain relief, if achieved, and the types of side effects, if they occurred. Then to complete step two, the nurses asked a hospice patient whose pain was under control to help them assign general levels of value to the sets of outcomes.

As a result of these activities, the nurses stated that they were more aware of the alternatives available to them. Also, they were able to describe the importance of identifying chance events over which they had no control and distinguishing those events from outcomes. In addition, the nurses indicated that the assignment of values to outcomes made them more conscious of patients' preferences and the significance of patient input into decision making.

The theoretical basis of decision analysis is decision theory, a mathematical, prescriptive model of decision making (Raiffa, 1968). Several assumptions are fundamental to this theory: (1) decisions are forms of risky choice made under conditions of uncertainty; (2) human beings make decisions rationally, that is, they select the alternative with the

Figure 1
A Decision Flow Diagram to Represent an Analgesic Dosage Titration Problem

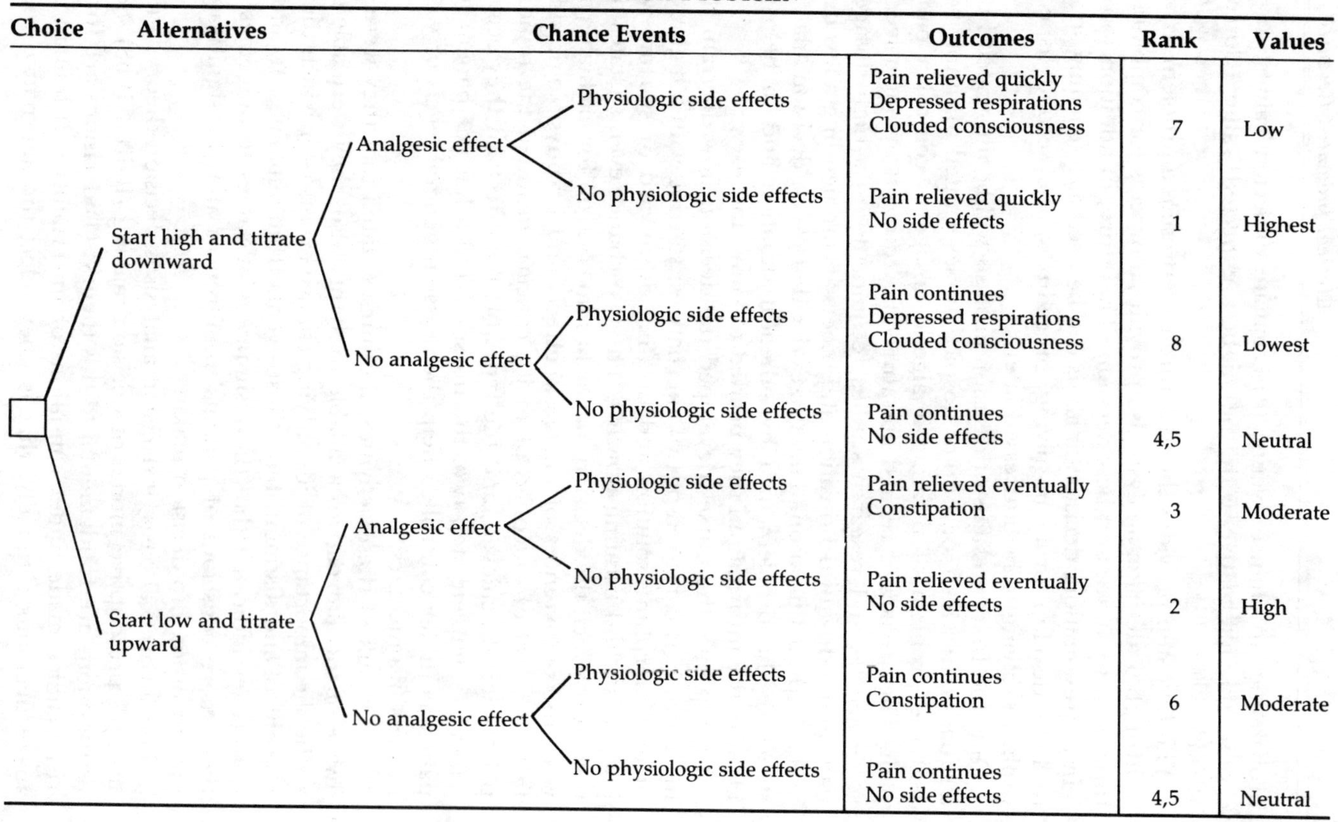

best outcome; and (3) estimates of probability and values must be independent of each other. Decision theory was used as the model of clinical judgment in studies by Grier (1976) and by Aspinall (1979) in which both researchers recommended instruction in formal decision theory as a means of improving clinical judgment performance.

Developing Problem-Solving Procedures

Two related instructional strategies can be used to help learners develop problem-solving strategies: iterative hypothesis testing and thinking aloud strategies.

Iterative Hypothesis Testing. As indicated in the literature review, recent research in nursing and in medicine provided evidence that clinicians use an iterative hypothesis testing strategy during diagnostic reasoning (Tanner, Padrick, Westfall, & Putzier, 1987; Elstein, Shulman, & Sprafka, 1978). The findings showed that clinicians: (1) formed diagnostic hypotheses based on minimal clinical data; (2) activated hypotheses very early in the process; and (3) used the activated hypotheses as a context for gathering additional relevant data to confirm or eliminate hypotheses. An iterative (repetitious) process was used. Kassirer (1983) suggested that such a process be used to teach diagnostic reasoning. The three phases of the strategy are: (1) asking questions to gather data about a patient; (2) justifying the data sought; and (3) interpreting the data to describe the new information's influence on decision making.

Iterative hypothesis testing will be illustrated in an inservice session with a group of telephone triage nurses in a seniors' clinic. The diagnostic task was to make a triage decision in a simulated situation. One nurse had worked with a patient who had called the clinic complaining of chest pain. That nurse served as a source of patient information as the other nurses collected data from him or her to decide about the appropriate disposition of the patient. The process of questioning, justifying, and interpreting occurred as follows.

After the nurse described the initial telephone conversation in which the patient complained of chest pain, another nurse began data collection by asking: "Where is the pain?" When asked to justify the question, the nurse who asked it indicated that he or she immediately thought of a myocardial infarction (MI) when he or she heard the complaint of chest pain and wanted more data to check that hypothesis. The group concurred with this justification. The nurse with the information stated that the patient's pain was substernal. Then the nurse who requested the data stated that the information was consistent with his or her hypothesis. This approach was continued as the next nurse asked for duration of pain with the rationale that he or she was pursuing classic symptoms of an MI. The response was that the pain had occurred on and off for the past two days. The nurse indicated that the new information did not fit the classic symptoms of MI and made him or her think of pulmonary embolus as an alternative hypothesis. The questioning, justifying, and interpreting continued as the nurses tested the competing hypotheses of MI and pulmonary embolus by gathering data about the intensity of pain, radiating pain, diaphoresis, and other associated symptoms. The group concluded the appropriate triage disposition was to send the paramedics to bring the patient into the emergency room (ER) to be seen by the physician because either condition could be a severe threat to life, threat being the basis for the triage decision. They also concluded that they actually needed very little information to make that decision, given the initial information of substernal chest pain. The nurse who had worked with the patient indicated that the patient was brought into the ER and had, in fact, suffered an MI.

The theoretical basis of this method is information processing theory which assumes that short-term memory has a limited capacity of seven plus or minus two chunks of information (Newell & Simon, 1972). The theory proposes that humans adapt to this limitation by collecting data selectively, processing data serially, and representing problems in simplified ways. In the iterative hypothesis testing strategy, the competing hypotheses guide the selection of data, based on the mental representations of the diagnostic conditions and their classic symptoms.

No reported studies have evaluated the effectiveness of iterative hypothesis testing as a teaching strategy. However, as described in the literature review, Tanner (1982) designed and tested a related experimental teaching method which focused on generating and testing diagnostic hypotheses. She found no significant main effects from the experimental treatment.

Thinking Aloud Strategy. Corcoran, Narayan, and Moreland (in press) proposed that since "thinking aloud" has been used successfully in research as a method for eliciting nurses' use of knowledge in clinical decision making, the strategy be used for instructional purposes as well. In this strategy a clinician is given a specific clinical situation and asked to "think aloud" while making a decision. The "thinking aloud" verbalizations are tape recorded and can later be transcribed, if desired. Analysis of such recordings or transcriptions reveals the information to which the clinician attends, the sequence in which information is processed, and the rules of thumb used to combine information and make decisions. From such data, inferences can be made about requisite factual knowledge, its structural organization, and practical knowledge gained through experience. This strategy is similar to iterative hypothesis testing, but it is less structured. In "thinking aloud" the nurses use their usual approaches instead of being required to question, justify, and interpret.

Thinking aloud can be used in peer dialogue among experienced nurses. To use this technique, nurses share their "thinking aloud" verbalizations, either formally or informally, to gain a better understanding of the knowledge they have and how they use it to arrive at diagnostic or treatment decisions about patients. To illustrate this process, refer again to the telephone triage nurses. Imagine that one nurse agrees to share data from an actual case and to serve as the repository of information about the patient. A second nurse offers to act as the triage nurse and "think aloud" while collecting data. The two nurses simulate a telephone triage interaction and tape record it while other nurses observe. Following the interaction, the tape recording is played back and stopped periodically as members of the group, including the participants, wish to comment on, or question interpretations of data, knowledge applied, and cognitive processes used. The nurse who brought the case reflects on the similarities and differences between his or her approach to the case and that of the nurse who thought aloud during the session. The discussion reveals rules of thumb used by the nurse, practical knowledge concerning variants of classic symptoms related to specific conditions, unique language used by the nurse to describe certain aspects of the case, and differences in approaches to telephone triage.

Another version of the "thinking aloud" strategy can serve nurses new to an area of practice, such as telephone triage, in different ways than it serves experienced nurses. For example, in telephone triage, new nurses need to understand the goal of triage and appreciate the distinction between a triage decision and a differential diagnosis. Also, they need guided experience to learn about the variants of textbook knowledge that are seen in practice and about rules of thumb. Support and feedback are necessary to facilitate the nurses' development. In one version of the strategy, an expert nurse might audiotape a simulated telephone triage interaction in which he or she "thinks aloud."

The expert then listens to the tape with a novice, reflecting on the expert's goal, the relevant issues in the case, how he or she elicited and interpreted data, the sequence in which he or she collected data, the rules he or she applied, and the arguments he or she used to arrive at a decision. The novice asks questions and clarifies his or her understanding of the expert's approach. In a second version of the strategy, a novice nurse might audiotape his or her simulated telephone triage interaction. Then, as the novice and mentor listen to the tape, they can stop it periodically for the novice to share his or her thinking at that point in the triage interaction. The mentor can reinforce the novice's appropriate use of knowledge and decision-making processes, and help him or her gain awareness of lack of knowledge or errors in thinking. The expert can emphasize the insights that can be achieved by examining errors as well as successes.

The theoretical basis of the thinking aloud strategy relates to information processing theory and the paradox of expertise described earlier (Newell & Simon, 1972; Johnson, 1983). Experts usually cannot describe how they perform tasks, but if asked to "think aloud" *while* doing the task much of their knowledge and cognitive processes can be revealed. The basis for suggesting "thinking aloud" as an instructional strategy is the belief that thinking aloud increases awareness of cognitive processes and, consequently, improves decision making. However, no empirical studies have been conducted to test the effectiveness of "thinking aloud" as an instructional strategy. Because much of the research on clinical judgment indicates the task-dependent and context-dependent nature of clinical decision making, few specific procedures can be identified which are generalizable across different types of cases. However, clinicians can identify the processes they use in specific situations, and then test those processes for effectiveness in similar cases.

Developing Pattern Recognition

Concept Attainment. Recognizing patterns or "chunks" of related pieces of information is one way of dealing with our limited short-term memory capacity. Frederiksen (1984) indicated that two ways of teaching pattern recognition are to provide opportunity for a great deal of practice and to model appropriate observational methods. However, another method does exist: concept attainment. By comparing positive and negative exemplars of a concept and extracting the essential attributes of the positive exemplars, one can learn the skills of classification and discrimination and develop broad concepts to serve as "chunks" of information. Then when one aspect of the concept or "chunk" is recalled, the related pieces of information are also recalled.

A teaching model for helping learners group data and form concepts is the Concept Attainment Model based on the work of Bruner, Goodnow, and Austin (1967). The learner is asked to place events or objects into classes by using certain cues and ignoring others. The learner discriminates relevant and irrelevant cues, generates and tests hypotheses, and groups data to form concepts. The three phases of the model are: (1) presenting data and identifying the concept; (2) testing attainment of the concept; and (3) analyzing thinking strategies (Joyce & Weil, 1986). This last phase of analyzing thinking strategies used a significant part of concept attainment and other models. Participants can "learn to learn" by reflecting on their cognitive strategies.

The following illustrates the Concept Attainment Model of teaching. Figure 2 contains a series of positive exemplars that contain the essential characteristics or attributes of a concept to be attained, as well as negative exemplars which do not represent the concept. Examine the exemplars and hypothesize what the concept is. Test the hypothesis(es) against each exemplar.

The concept is change. The attributes of the positive exemplars include: (1) something is altered; (2) a process occurs over time; (3) the direction of the alteration is either forward or backward; and (4) the alteration may or may not involve identity. The critical attribute is that something is altered. The other attributes may or may not be present

Figure 2
Positive and Negative Exemplars for Attainment of a Specific Concept

Positive Exemplars	Negative Exemplars
A pencil is 6½ inches long. After use, it is 4 inches long.	A pencil is 6½ inches long. After one week, it still is 6½ inches long.
A cocoon sits on a branch. A few days later it opens and a beautiful butterfly appears.	A man smokes 2 packs of cigarettes a day. At the end of a Stop Smoking course, he still smokes 2 packs a day.
A child speaks in clear, complete sentences. After the birth of a sibling, she starts using baby talk and single words.	A woman in a weight control class maintains her weight at 125 lbs.

in positive exemplars; therefore, they are not critical. For example, the attribute of period of time is included in both positive and negative exemplars; therefore, it is not critical or essential. Next one could test attainment of the concept by having students generate their own positive exemplars. The final step is to analyze the thinking strategies used in the process of categorizing and attaining the concept. Is it worth the time required to attain concepts in this way? It depends on the importance of the concept and on the value placed on developing thinking skills of discrimination, categorization, and pattern recognition.

The concept attainment model can be very useful in clarifying major concepts within the discipline of nursing. It could be an effective model for clarifying nursing diagnoses and their defining characteristics. Concept attainment could also be an alternative to traditional clinical laboratory activities. Suppose students are to learn the concept of immobility with its associated side effects and possible complications. Nursing rounds could be arranged so that students interact with patients who are experiencing a variety of conditions that are associated with immobility, such as a comatose patient, a patient with a fractured hip who is on a circle bed, an elderly patient who is in restraints, and an infant who has not developed the ability to move independently. These patients could be contrasted with patients who are mobile. Then students could extract the essential attributes of immobility and design related nursing interventions. There has been extensive research on the development of concepts, primarily with children as subjects. However, the findings which support this model seem to apply equally well to adults.

To summarize, we have just examined: (a) two teaching strategies for developing problem representation, analogies and decision analysis; (b) two strategies for developing problem-solving procedures, iterative hypothesis testing and thinking aloud strategies; and (c) one strategy for developing pattern recognition, concept attainment. These instructional strategies are useful in individual class sessions. Now we will turn to consideration of several implications of clinical judgment research for curricular planning.

IMPLICATIONS FOR CURRICULUM PLANNING

Clinical judgment research findings have implications for curriculum content, sequence, and methods. Students need a broad knowledge base in content from their support courses to serve as a foundation for qualitative and quantitative aspects of clinical decision making. A breadth of coursework from the humanities, as well as from the behavioral, natural, and health sciences is needed to develop a perspective of patients as whole persons and of health as a broad concept. For example, clinical decision making can easily focus attention on only particular problems or specific aspects of a person, so students need a holistic perspective to relate the particular decision task to the whole person and to involve the person in the decision process. From a quantitative perspective, coursework in mathematics, including probability theory, is prerequisite to understanding and applying decision theory. In addition, knowledge of probability theory helps students become aware of the uncertainty that exists in most nursing situations. Also, it can promote more complete and accurate recording of clinical data because students learn to appreciate the importance of aggregate data and objective probabilities for predicting likely chance events and outcomes associated with their decisions and actions.

Findings from clinical judgment research have implications for curriculum sequence, too. Benner's (1984) studies show that novices are rule-based decision makers. They have little clinical experience to support their judgments, so they must rely on acontextual rules. Therefore, it is appropriate to provide such acontextual rules early in the nursing curriculum. However, as students progress in the program, they should be encouraged to challenge and test the acontextual rules, and to identify and examine the practical knowledge they are developing in their clinical experiences. Also, as students progress, they are able to interact more effectively with expert clinicians as their experience enables them to understand the language experts use to describe their perceptual knowledge, language which novices usually cannot comprehend. The essential point here is this: do not rely on a single method of teaching (as we have traditionally done with the nursing care plan) to teach students across all levels.

Finally, findings from clinical judgment research have implications for curriculum methods, including the specific teaching strategies previously described, as well as general learning activities. Both faculty and students need to develop a repertoire of approaches to clinical reasoning. The nursing process alone is no longer adequate. In the past it served nursing well by emphasizing the scientific method and its relevance to nursing. However, the steps of the nursing process are too general to be useful in actual practice. In addition, research findings indicate that nurses do not use a linear process, nor are their cognitive processes invariant across decision-making tasks. It is important to give students time and guidance to reflect on their own thinking processes and to compare their processes with those of peers and more experienced nurses.

CONCLUSION

Findings from clinical judgment research have implications for teaching and for curriculum planning in nursing education. We have identified underlying assumptions, briefly reviewed the research literature on clinical judgment, and identified implications. It is an exciting time to be involved in nursing education. The developing field of cognitive science and the ongoing work in decision theory and phenomenology, along with the growing body of research regarding clinical decision making are beginning to come together to provide meaningful guidance for nursing clinicians and educators.

REFERENCES

Alexander, P., White, C. S., Haensley, P., & Crimmins-Jeanes, M. (1987). Training in analogical reasoning. *American Educational Research Journal, 24*(3), 387–404.

Aspinall, M. J. (1979). Use of a decision tree to improve accuracy of diagnosis. *Nursing Research, 28*, 182–185.

Benner, P. (1984). *From novice to expert: Excellence and power in clinical nursing practice*. Menlo Park, CA: Addison-Wesley.

Bruner, J., Goodnow, J., & Austin, G. (1967). *A study of thinking*. New York: Wiley.

Corcoran, S. (1986a). Task complexity and nursing expertise as factors in decision making. *Nursing Research, 35*(2), 107–112.

Corcoran, S. (1986b). Decision analysis: A guide for decision making in clinical nursing. *Nursing and Health Care, 7*(3), 148–154.

Corcoran, S., Narayan, S., & Moreland, H. (in press). Thinking aloud as a strategy to improve clinical decision making. *Journal of Professional Nursing*.

Davis, B. G. (1972). Clinical expertise as a function of educational preparation. *Nursing Research, 21*, 530–534.

Davis, B. G. (1974). Effect of levels of nursing education on patient care: A replication. *Nursing Research, 23*, 150–155.

del Bueno, D. J. (1983). Doing the right thing: Nurses' ability to make clinical decisions. *Nurse Educator, 8*(3), 7–11.

deTornyay, R. (1968a). The effect of an experimental teaching strategy on problem solving abilities of sophomore nursing students. *Nursing Research, 17*, 108–114.

deTornyay, R. (1968b). Measuring problem-solving skills by means of the simulated clinical nursing problems test. *Journal of Nursing Education, 5*(8), 3–8.

Dincher, J. R., & Stidger, S. L. (1976). Evaluation of a written simulation format for clinical nursing judgment: A pilot study. *Nursing Research, 25*, 280–285.

Elstein, A., Shulman, L., & Sprafka, S. (1978). *Medical problem solving*. Cambridge, MA: MIT Press.

Frederiksen, N. (1984). Implications of cognitive theory for instruction in problem solving. *Review of Educational Research, 54*(3), 363–407.

Frederickson, K., & Mayer, G. G. (1977). Problem solving skills, What effect does education have? *American Journal of Nursing, 77*, 1167–1169.

Gordon, W. (1970). *The metaphorical way of learning and knowing*. Cambridge, MA: Synectics Education Press.

Gordon, M. (1980). Predictive strategies in diagnostic tasks. *Nursing Research, 29*, 39–45.

Grier, M. (1976). Decision making about patient care. *Nursing Research, 25*(2), 105–110.

Holyoak, K. J. (1984). Analogical thinking and human intelligence. In R. J. Sternberg (ed.). *Advances in the psychology of human intelligence: Vol. 2* (pp. 199–230). Hillsdale, NJ: Lawrence Erlbaum.

Holzemer, W. (1986). The structure of problem solving in simulations. *Nursing Research, 35*, 231–236.

Holzemer, W. L., Schleutermann, J. A., Farrand, L., & Miller, A. G. (1981). A validation study: Simulations as a measure of nurse practitioners' problem-solving skills. *Nursing Research, 30*, 139–144.

Johnson, P. E. (1983). What kind of an expert should a system be? *Journal of Medicine and Philosophy, 8*, 77–97.

Joyce, B., & Weil, M. (1986). *Models of teaching* (3rd ed.). Englewood Cliffs, NJ: Prentice-Hall.

Kassirer, J. (1983). Sounding board: Teaching clinical medicine by iterative hypothesis testing. *New England Journal of Medicine, 309*(15), 921–924.

Koehne-Kaplan, N. S., & Tilden, V. P. (1976). The process of clinical judgment in nursing practice: The component of personality. *Nursing Research, 25*, 268–272.

McIntyre, H. N., McDonalia, F. J., Bailey, J. T., & Claus, K. K. (1972). A simulated clinical nursing test. *Nursing Research, 21*, 429–435.

McLaughlin, F. E., Carr, J., & Delucchi, K. (1981). Measurement properties of clinical simulation tests: Hypertension and chronic obstructive pulmonary disease. *Nursing Research, 30*, 5–9.

Mitchell, P. H., & Atwood, J. (1975). Problem-oriented recording as a teaching learning tool. *Nursing Research, 24*, 99–103.

Newell, A., & Simon, H. (1972). *Human problem solving*. Englewood Cliffs, NJ: Prentice-Hall.

Pyles, S. H., & Stern, P. N. (1983). Discovery of nursing gestalt in critical care nursing: The importance of the gray gorilla syndrome. *Image: The Journal of Nursing Scholarship, 15*(2), 51–57.

Raiffa, H. (1968). *Decision analysis: Introductory lectures on choice under uncertainty.* Reading, MA: Addison-Wesley.

Simon, H. (1979). Information processing models of cognition. *Annual Review of Psychology, 30,* 363–396.

Sternberg, R. J. (1983). Criteria for intellectual skills training. *Educational Researcher, 12*(2), 6–13.

Tanner, C. (1982). Instruction in the diagnostic process: An experimental study. In M. J. Kim & D. Moritz (Eds.), *Classification of Nursing Diagnoses: Proceedings of the Third and Fourth National Conferences* (pp. 145–152.) New York: McGraw-Hill.

Tanner, C., Padrick, K., Westfall, U., & Putzier, D. (1987). diagnostic reasoning strategies of nurses and nursing students. *Nursing Research, 36*(6), 358–363.

Tanner, C. (1987). Teaching clinical judgment. In J. J. Fitzpatrick & R. L. Tauton (Eds.), *Annual Review of Nursing Research, Vol. 5,* New York: pp. 153–173.

Westfall, U., Tanner, C., Putzier, D., & Padrick, K. (1986). Activating clinical inferences: A component of diagnostic reasoning in nursing. *Research in Nursing and Health, 9,* 269–277.

Verhonick, P. J., Nichols, G. A., Glor, B. A. K., & McCarthy, R. T. (1968). I came, I saw, I responded: Nursing observation and action survey. *Nursing Research, 17,* 38–44.

11

Curriculum Outcomes and Cognitive Development: New Perspectives for Nursing Education

Theresa M. Valiga

WHY BE CONCERNED ABOUT CURRICULUM OUTCOMES?

The quest for quality in higher education is nothing new. Since its inception, the higher educational system has been concerned with transmitting the knowledge and values of a given culture, with generating and testing new knowledge, with helping students to think critically and to learn how to learn, and with fostering the total development of the student. These goals have been the cornerstone of higher education for centuries. Recently, however, questions have been raised about our educational systems by people within and outside the profession, and grave concerns about the quality of education and the capabilities of its graduates have been expressed. Although nursing education has not been the center of such criticism—indeed, it has not even been singled out in texts on quality and excellence in education—we cannot think that it does not apply to us.

I contend that nurse educators must be as sensitive to the criticisms of educational outcomes as professors of sociology, physics, and history are—perhaps even more sensitive, in light of the far-reaching changes in our society and our health care systems with which nurses must be concerned. Imagine a society characterized by the following:

- scarce resources and increased competition;
- increased collaboration and interdependence (or, as Luther Christman called it, an increase in "operational alliances");
- decreased territoriality and the maintenance of a world view rather than a narrow national or regional view;
- increased politicization and involvement of consumers in decision making and policy setting;
- increased diversity and pluralism;
- temporariness, fluidity, and constant change;
- increased individualism;
- enthusiasm for the unknown ambiguity;
- an increased range of options (or, as Martha Rogers puts it, "a shifting panorama of infinite possibilities") ;
- increased self-care and self-responsibility, accompanied by increased consumer sophistication;
- more and more complex technology;
- population shifts and the development of a four-generation society;
- more difficult ethical dilemmas;
- less materialism and greater emphasis on the value of human relationships and intangibles;
- greater decentralization;
- diverse employment patterns, with work becoming more intellectually demanding and increasingly motivated by worker's need for personal growth and self-development; and
- continuing knowledge explosion, coupled with increased demand for more advanced educational preparation.

Such a society may seem an exciting prospect, and perhaps a frightening one as well. In fact, however, it is essentially the society we live in now and will continue to live in for some time. If we, as educators, are responsible for preparing nurses to function in and shape this society, we cannot ignore the ever more widespread concerns being expressed with respect to educational excellence and educational outcomes. Several recent expressions of concern deserve brief review here.

RECENT EXPRESSIONS OF CONCERN

A few years ago, the Study Group on the Conditions of Excellence in American Higher Education (1984) published an important report. Working from the belief that the United States should be a nation of educated people who are knowledgeable, creative, and open to ideas and who have "learned how to learn so they can pursue knowledge throughout their lives and assist their children in the same quest" (p. 35), the Study Group asserted that "higher learning in America should be broadened and deepened so as to provide increased opportunities for intellectual, cultural and personal growth of all our citizens" (p. 35).

The Study Group also concluded that institutions of higher education must produce demonstrable improvements in student knowledge, capacities, skills, and attitudes between entrance and graduation. They suggested that such demonstrable improvements could be achieved through (1) significantly increasing student involvement in the learning process; (2) setting, publicizing, and maintaining high expectations for student performance, thereby minimizing the extent to which educators underestimate students and fail to help them reach their potentials; and (3) providing regular, personalized, meaningful, critical, and constructive assessment and feedback.

Futhermore, the Study Group urged that first- and second-year students receive the greatest amount of faculty and university resources, since it is in the first two years that students are most open, most receptive, and most likely to grow and change significantly. Finally, they argued that "all bachelor's degree recipients should have at least two full years of liberal education [which] in most professional fields . . . will require extending undergraduate programs beyond the usual four years" (p. 43). Such recommendations certainly give nurse educators food for thought.

A second major report was published by the Association of American Colleges' Project on Redefining the Meaning and Purpose of Baccalaureate Degrees (1985). This report was concerned with "integrity in the college curriculum" and was undertaken because of "the decline and devaluation of the undergraduate degree" (p. 12). The project panel observed that "the major in most colleges is little more than a gathering of courses taken in one department, lacking structure and depth . . . or emphasizing content to the neglect of the essential style of inquiry on which the content is based" (p. 21).

I would not argue that nursing programs lack structure and depth

—indeed, they are sometimes so structured and rigid that they become highly restrictive. I would, however, argue that nursing programs often focus so much on the content that they lose sight of process and outcomes. We sometimes seem to assume that if we give our students enough content—that is, enough facts, principles, and information—they will automatically learn how to process that information and make decisions regarding nursing practice and will automatically develop the set of values we would want them to have as they assume positions of professional nurses in our society. To my mind, this assumption is questionable at best.

The AAC project panel also proposed a "minimum required program of study for all students that . . . consists of 'the intellectual, esthetic, and philosophic experiences that should enter into the lives of men and women engaged in baccalaureate education'" (p. 13). This program would aim at developing the following:

- literacy (namely, writing, reading, speaking and listening at a level of distinction);
- an understanding of numerical data, which enables students to provide "a sophisticated response to arguments and positions which depend on numbers and statistics" (p. 19);
- a historical consciousness;
- an understanding of the scientific method and the "human, social, and political implications of scientific research" (p. 20);
- a value system that encourages students to "make real choices, assume responsibility for their decisions, be comfortable with their own behavior, and know why" (p. 20);
- an understanding of the language of fine arts;
- "insights and understandings [of] the lives and aspirations of the distant and foreign, the different and neglected" (p. 22)—that is, those of different cultures and different worlds;
- skills of inquiry, abstract logical thinking and critical analysis, which enables students to "reason well . . . recognize when reason and evidence are not enough . . . [and] discover the legitimacy of intuition" (p. 18); and
- a depth of knowledge that leads to "more sophisticated understanding and encourages leaps of the imagination and efforts at synthesis" (p. 22).

No doubt many nurse educators, having read this list, will think to themselves, "We already do all that." Not long ago, I would have had the same reaction. But the more carefully I looked at what was actually being accomplished in baccalaureate programs, the more I talked with the faculty who teach in those programs about what they do, and the more I found out about the knowledge, skills, abilities, and values of the students in and graduates of such programs, the more I began to question this view. I believe that if we are honest with ourselves, we will have to admit that our educational system has some significant deficiencies that must be addressed.

Another important report was published by the Carnegie Foundation for the Advancement of Teaching (1985). Taking into account the growing complexity of the world, the truly international perspective we now must employ, and the continuing tightening of resources, the Foundation called for a thorough examination of "whether [our] current programs and policies are achieving their educational and scholarly goals" (p. 17) and proposed that we undertake "a period of purposeful renewal" (p. 17).

While conceding that a career and an understanding of technology are important to today's graduates, the Foundation asserted that other things are, or should be, just as important: "the capacity to take initiative, to be creative, to understand the international nature of the world, and to comprehend the need to both compete and cooperate" (p. 20). Such abilities, it argued, are critical if we are to meet "the formidable tasks ahead" (p. 20). Finally, the Foundation concluded, we need graduates who have a greater sense of public purpose and civic-mindedness and are less caught up in self-interest and parochialism.

Last year, two books appeared that questioned the effectiveness of our educational systems (Bloom, 1987; Ravitch & Finn, 1987) In *The Closing of the American Mind* (which is subtitled *How Higher Education Has Failed Democracy and Impoverished the Souls of Today's Students*), Bloom contends that "attention to the young, knowing what their hungers are and what they can digest, is the essence of the craft [of teaching]" (p. 19). He asserts that the truly educated person is the one who, in our "chronic lack of certainty" (p. 21), knows alternatives and thinks about them, who resists the "easy and preferred answers, not because he is obstinate but because he knows others worthy of consideration" (p. 21), and who is open. Indeed, according to Bloom, "the only danger confronting us is being *closed* to the emergent, the new, the manifestations of progress" (p. 29).

Unfortunately, Bloom concludes, today's students know much less, are much more cut off from tradition, and are "much slacker intellectually" (p. 51) than their predecessors; moreover, they have "lost the practice of and the taste for reading" (p. 62). But the fault does not rest only with them: it also rests with our culture, with our educational system, and with us as faculty.

Lack of commitment to a liberal education closes students' minds. Professors who are specialists, concerned only with their own fields or with their own personal advancement, close students' minds. Failure to recognize and discuss important questions of common concern closes students' minds. All these things should be anathema to educators. Our job is to open minds, not to close them.

Ravitch and Finn (1987) also question the quality of our educational systems, but from a different perspective. This book is a report of a research study that assessed the level of knowledge of history and literature attained by nearly 8,000 17-year-olds. As the makeup of the population might suggest, the book does not make specific recommendations with respect to higher education; nevertheless, I believe that its conclusions are indeed relevant to higher education.

Ravitch and Finn (1987) found that high school juniors, despite having progressed through a variety of educational experiences, have a poor knowledge of both history (only 54 percent of the most basic history questions were answered correctly) and literature (only 52 percent of the most basic literature questions were answered correctly). Overall, 29 clusters of questions were asked. The group received a grade of F in 20 of them, a grade of D minus in 5, a grade of D in 1, a grade of D plus in 1, and a grade of C minus in 2. The group did not receive a single B or A.

Is it possible that the same situation is present in higher educational settings as well? Could it be that some students—perhaps far too many students—pass through four years of baccalaureate education without really learning all they should or could learn? How many students may have received a degree without receiving an education?

WHAT OUTCOMES DO WE WANT?

Undoubtedly, these recent reports have raised serious questions about what we educators are doing in our educational programs and what the products or outcomes of higher education are. Are the outcomes we are achieving the ones we really want?

Nurse educators must ask these same questions. What is going on in our nursing programs? Are we truly concerned with the total development of our students—as professional nurses, as citizens, and as human beings—or are we concerned only with delivering content? Are we so obsessed with being in control that we stifle our students' creativity and ability to think critically? Are we truly encouraging our students to be skeptical and inquisitive, or are we—whether subtly or openly—promoting the attitude that there is one right way to do things? Finally, are we excellent role models, not just as competent practitioners of nursing but also as individuals with a broad and diverse (rather than a narrow and limited) perspective? As civic-minded individuals? As people who are open to new ideas and approaches? As nurses who write, speak, and listen at a level of distinction? Are we able to reason well but are we also comfortable with intuition? Are we imaginative, creative, and willing to take initiative? Are we involved professionally and committed to our work? Are we willing to set high expectations for ourselves and others and to invest ourselves in ensuring that these expectations are achieved? Are we this kind of role model, and are we producing this kind of graduate?

In a recent annotated bibliography published by the NLN (1987), Sylvia Hart noted that "assessment of educational outcomes and accountability for the quality of the products of educational programs are interrelated concepts that have become increasingly important in recent years" (p. v). She advised the nursing profession in particular to take pains to ensure that "program quality [is] systematically monitored, measured, and documented" (p. v). In her view, "the results of reliable and valid measures of students' knowledge, attitudes, and performances upon completion of an educational program, especially in a practice-based profession such as nursing, are essential if decisions regarding the program's quality and effectiveness are to be tenable" (p. ix). If we accept this view, we must expand our focus, which currently embraces only the antecedents to and processes within our programs, to include the outcomes of our programs. This is the thrust of the Accreditation Outcomes Project, now being conducted by the NLN with funding from the Helene Fuld Health Trust.

One important question remains: precisely what are the educational outcomes to which we need to attend? Clearly they include such things as academic achievement (as assessed by measures such as grades, grade point averages, and performance on standardized tests), program completion versus attrition rates, clinical performance, evaluation of graduates by employers, and the success of graduates in their careers. Perhaps less obviously, they also include empathy, verbal and written communication skills, logical problem solving, decision making, moral reasoning, ethical decision making, professional attitudes and socialization, self-concept, self-esteem, confidence, values, and leadership and followership abilities. The major areas of development that have been advocated or documented as a result of higher education are cognitive development, flexibility, creativity, openness to experience, responsibility, intellectual tolerance, sense of self, other-centeredness, judgment, the ability to make independent yet informed decisions, autonomy (self-directed behavior), and integrated and consistent values. In the remainder of this chapter, I will concentrate on one of these, namely, cognitive development.

COGNITIVE DEVELOPMENT AS AN EDUCATIONAL OUTCOME

Those of us who have spent many years writing objectives probably think automatically of the cognitive domain when the term *cognitive development* is mentioned. By and large, we probably feel that we do address cognitive development in nursing education programs. I would not disagree with this belief; however, I think we need to remind ourselves that the concept of cognitive development embraces far more than mere comprehension, analysis, synthesis, and evaluation. It also includes all of the following:

- ability to be comfortable with conceptual complexity;
- ability to tolerate ambiguity and uncertainty;
- ability to manage diversity and conflicting information;
- ability to make decisions despite incomplete and fallible information;
- ability to reason clearly;
- ability to arrive at a concise, informed synthesis of the critical issues involved in a situation;
- ability to structure and organize knowledge and experience;
- ability to reason in an open and critical fashion;
- ability to behave flexibly;
- ability to take in other views while retaining one's own;
- ability to take on new roles; and
- ability to use criticism in creative achievement.

Cognitive (or intellectual) development, then, is defined in terms of increasingly complex cognitive skills, not in terms of verbal and mathematical skills measured by aptitude or achievement tests, and not in terms of isolated traits such as rationality, critical thinking, intellectual tolerance, and creativity. Briefly put, cognitive development is how individuals reason about issues and, in particular, how they take diverse viewpoints into consideration. Ways of encouraging the development of the skills listed above is a legitimate concern for nurse educators, since one of the most significant purposes of college, as Kurfiss (1975) says, is to provide students with the "cognitive weapons for the battle with diversity" (p. 75). Surely very few of us have to be convinced diversity is a major characteristic of the nursing profession.

Much of the work that has been done on cognitive development is based on that of Piaget, who outlined four stages of cognitive development and asserted that the process of development of cognitive schemata begins at birth and culminates in adolescence. This line of thinking has been challenged by many experts who have offered alternative ideas about lifelong development. One of these challengers is Perry (1970), whose ideas I will discuss in some detail. Before describing Perry's model, however, I must first list some important characteristics of cognitive development:

- it occurs in stages;
- the stages are sequential, predictable, and progressive;
- each stage incorporates and expands on elements of the previous stage; and
- it is impossible to "go back" all the way (an idea similar to Martha Rogers' concept of unidirectionality).

Perry did his original research at Harvard in the middle to late 1950s. His subjects were all male liberal arts students. He asked them to discuss their educational experiences at the start of their freshman year, and at the end of the freshman, sophmore, junior, and senior years. The discussions were free-flowing and open-ended. From the comments made in them, Perry developed a nine-position scheme that reflected development in two different domains, the epistemological and the ethical.

The dominant themes in the Perry scheme are the nature of knowledge and the individual's relationship to authority. Other themes are decision making or judgment, simplicity versus complexity, right versus wrong, responsibility, the nature of reasoning, the use of evidence, an open versus a closed perspective, varying explanations of differences in viewpoint, and concreteness versus abstractness.

Perry's nine positions are divided into three general categories: dualism, relativism, and commitment in relativism. These positions and categories are summarized in Table 1.

Table 1
Perry's Main Line of Cognitive Development*

Dualism

The first three positions represent a view of the world of knowledge as dualistic. The learner views himself as a receptacle ready to receive truth; as a result, he has difficulty with academic tasks requiring recognition of conflicting points of view or use of his own position (Knefelkamp, 1974, p. 18).

Position 1: The student sees the world in polar terms of we-right-good vs. other-wrong-bad. Right answers for everything exist in the absolute, known to authority, whose role is to mediate (teach) them.

Position 2: The student perceives diversity of opinion and uncertainty, and accounts for them as unwarranted confusion in poorly qualified authorities or as mere exercises set by authority "so we can learn to find the answer for ourselves."

Position 3: The student accepts diversity and uncertainty as legitimate but still temporary in areas where authority "hasn't found the answer yet." He supposes authority grades him in these areas on "good expression," but remains puzzled as to standards.

Relativism

Positions 4, 5, and 6 describe movement to recognition of knowledge as relative. In this sequence, "truth" is first relegated to a small corner of the broader realm of knowledge, which is uncertain. Then, with position 5, all knowledge and values are disconnected from the concept of truth or absolute correctness. In a sense, with relativism of knowlege may come loss of the old signposts and the experience of being lost and alone in a chaotic world. Yet movement along positions 4, 5, and 6 creates an awareness that much of what "truth" he "creates" will emerge from the student's own experience and judgment as well as external factors (Knefelkamp, 1974, p. 19).

Position 4: (a) The student perceives legitimate uncertainty (and therefore diversity of opinion) to be extensive and raises it to the status of an unstructured epistemologic realm of its own in which "anyone has a right to his own opinion," a realm that he sets over against authority's realm, where right-wrong still prevails; or (b) the student discovers qualitative contextual relativistic reasoning as a special case of "what they want" within authority's realm.

Position 5: The student perceives all knowledge and values (including authority's) as contextual and relativistic and subordinates dualistic right-wrong functions to the status of a special case, in context.

Position 6: The student apprehends the necessity of orienting himself in a relativistic world through some form of personal commitment (as distinct from unquestioned or unconsidered commitment to simple belief in certainty).

Commitment in Relativism

During positions 7, 8, and 9, the student gradually accepts the responsibility of the pluralistic world and acts through commitment to establish his identity. There are two components to commitment. First is a coming to terms with the content of one's commitment by selecting a particular career, a set of values, a marriage partner. The other aspect appears to be based upon the individual's recognition that within himself are many diverse, conflicting personal themes (Knefelkamp, 1974, p. 20).

Position 7: The student makes an initial commitment in some area.

Position 8: The student experiences the implications of commitment and explores the subjective and stylistic issues of responsibility.

Position 9: The student experiences the affirmation of identity among multiple responsibilities and realizes commitment as an ongoing, unfolding activity through which he expresses his life style.

*Drawn from Perry (1970, pp. 9–10).

Essentially, the dualistic view of the world is very narrow; authority is very sure, and truth and "the right behavior" are easily determined. The relativistic view accepts more options. A person who has arrived at commitment in relativism rejects or chooses not to consider some of the options accepted by the relativistic view, but only after careful consideration and evaluation of alternatives.

Once we have some understanding of what cognitive development is, we need to know what prompts it. Most cognitive development models suggest that development results from disequilibrium. When people are faced with information that cannot be assimilated into their existing structure, they change that structure to make it admit more complexity. Cognitive developmental theory even suggests that contact with diversity is necessary to motivate people to break with old frames of reference and that diverse experiences are necessary to promote development to higher levels (Figure 1). We should ask ourselves whether nurses in practice and students in educational settings are really being exposed to significant diversity.

Research on Cognitive Development

Most of the research related to the Perry scheme has focused on the educational environment. This focus arises from (1) the belief that the process of development, of progression through stages, is interactional and (2) the belief that development requires both readiness within the individual and stimulation from the environment. Studies using the

Figure 1
Process of Change in Developmental Position*

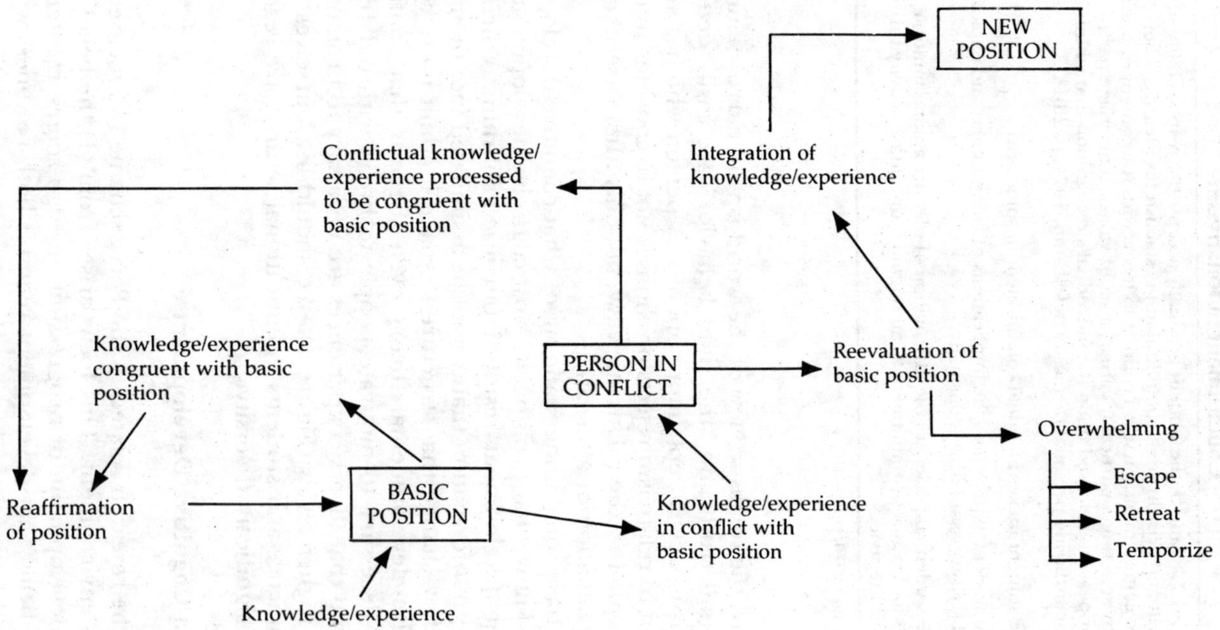

*Adapted from Cordts (1977).

Perry scheme have related cognitive development to a number of variables, including

- the degree of structure and flexibility provided;
- the nature of peer interactions among students;
- the openness of student-faculty relationships;
- the degree of challenge and support provided;
- the types of course assignments given;
- the extent to which the learning environment is "matched" with the student's position;
- age;
- gender;
- socioeconomic status;
- verbal fluency;
- the size of the student's home town (as a measure of homogeneity);
- the student's motives for pursuing education;
- the student's preference for a learning style; and
- the type of curriculum (i.e., liberal arts or science) in which the student was enrolled.

Some of the findings of these studies should be of interest to nurse educators. Knefelkamp (1974) studied the impact of the educational environment on students' cognitive development. She found that 28 of 31 students in a one-semester course gained in Perry position, and many of them gained almost a full position.

Widick (1975) studied the relationships between students' Perry position and the types of assignments they preferred or did better on and between position and the focus of the classroom. She found that 90 percent of the students in a one-semester course gained in Perry position and that 75 percent of this group gained at least 0.5 position. She also found that relativistic students did better with take-home essays (because these require more complex skills) and that dualistic students did better on short-answer tests (because these tend to be more objective-oriented).

Touchton, Wertheimer, Cornfeld, and Harrison (1977) evaluated movement in Perry position in (1) classes taught in a traditional (i.e., teacher-controlled) way, (2) classes taught with developmental instruction methods, and (3) classes taught in a mixed way (i.e., taught traditionally but by a teacher with knowledge of developmental theory). They found that only 41 percent of the students in the traditional class gained in position, whereas 65 percent of those in the mixed class and 76 percent of those in the developmental instruction class gained in position.

Generally, studies in this area have shown that (1) age, by itself, makes no difference in Perry position; (2) students from small home towns come from more homogeneous backgrounds and show a smaller range of scores and lower scores overall; (3) abstract conceptualizations and reflective thought are preferred by men, traditional-age students, and freshmen; and (4) concrete conceptualizations and active experimentation are preferred by women, adult learners, and seniors.

Nurses who engage in professional practice must be able to combine theoretical and empirical knowledge from various disciplines with nursing knowledge. Unfortunately, the knowledge offered by these various disciplines is often limited, or conflicting, or both, which means that nurses must know how to evaluate the knowledge available, be aware of its evolutionary status, and be able to reach some decision about its usefulness in specific practice situations. It would seem, therefore, that if nurses are to engage in truly professional practice, they must be able to deal effectively with uncertainty. Schein (1972) maintains that this ability is a hallmark of the professional.

> An important part of the training of a professional is what some sociologists have called "training for uncertainty" . . . which involves . . . components such as [1] maintenance of one's self-confidence even when one does not have a clear answer to the problem, [2] willingness to take responsibility for key decisions that may rest on only partial information, [3] willingness to make a decision under conditions of high risk, [4] the ability to inspire confidence in the client even when operating in an area of high uncertainty, and so on. (pp. 44–45)

Professional nurses also are expected to assume responsibility, to be self-directive, to be introspective, to be able to analyze and synthesize data, to be able to deal with multiple perspectives, to be able to define their nursing role and articulate it clearly to clients and other professionals, and to take risks with themselves. I believe that if nurses are to fulfill these expectations, they must be at more advanced stages of cognitive development (Figure 2).

I undertook a study designed to determine how much progress nursing students made with respect to cognitive development over the

Figure 2
A Process Model of Human Development: Areas of Qualitative Change*

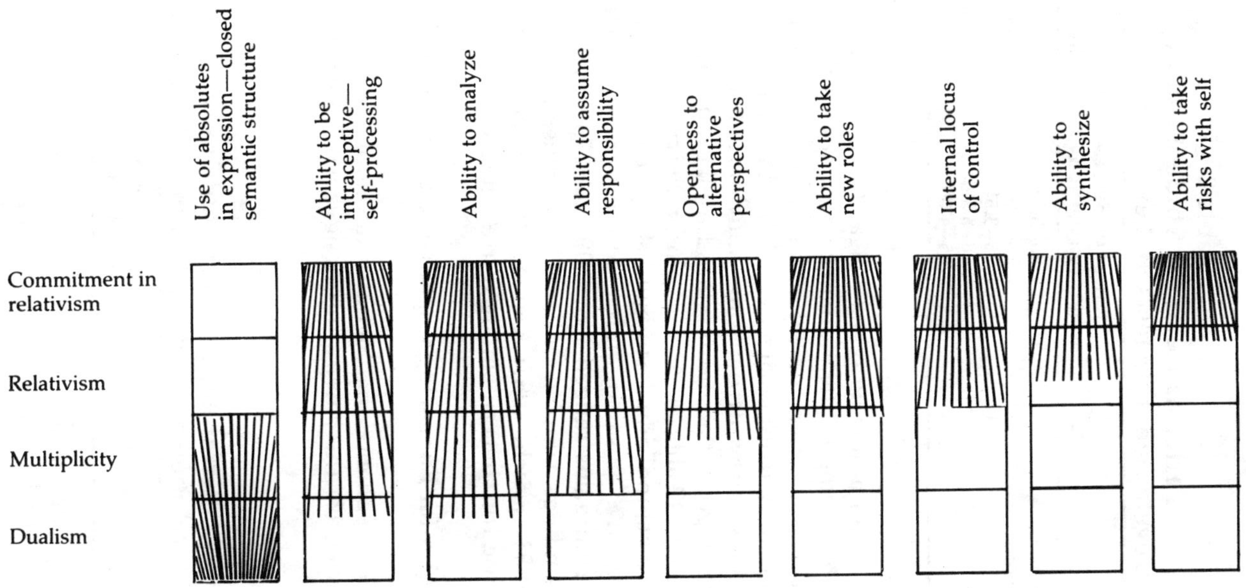

Degree of density corresponds with degree to which variable is present.

*Adapted from Knefelkamp and Slepitza (1976).

Table 2
Performance of 123 Students on Cognitive Development Pretests by Level of Nursing Education

Level	N	Range of Scores (Perry Position)	Mean	Standard Deviation
Freshman	29	2.25–3.25	2.73	.272
Sophomore	27	2.58–4.00	3.06	.424
Junior	34	2.25–3.58	2.96	.294
Senior	33	2.58–3.92	3.10	.338
Total	123	2.25–4.00	2.96	.359

course of an academic year (Valiga, 1982; Valiga, 1983). I found that at the beginning of the academic year, most of the 123 students tested were dualistic on an individual basis; the means for all groups clearly fell into the dualistic category (Table 2). At the end of the academic year, the same was true: some individuals had progressed to the relativistic stage, but all mean scores for all groups still fell into the dualistic category (Table 3). As for gains in Perry position over the academic year, some individual students showed no change, some gained as much as 1.75 position, and some regressed as much as 1.50 position. The mean gains ranged from .091 to .275 position (Table 4). Surely these findings, coupled with similar findings from other research (Collins, 1981; Frisch, 1987; Kiener, 1984; Sakalys, 1984; Watson, 1978), are cause for concern among nurse educators.

Strategies for Enhancing Cognitive Development

We can enhance the cognitive development of nursing students by improving (1) the curriculum designs we implement, (2) the teaching

Table 3
Performance of 123 Students on Cognitive Development Posttests by Level of Nursing Education

Level	N	Range of Scores (Perry Position)	Mean	Standard Deviation
Freshman	29	2.25–3.67	2.82	.350
Sophomore	27	2.33–5.08	3.18	.672
Junior	34	2.42–4.17	3.05	.419
Senior	33	2.08–5.59	3.41	.730
Total	123	2.08–5.59	3.12	.597

Table 4
Degree of Change in Cognitive Development Scores Manifested by 123 Students From Fall to Spring

Level	Change	*P*
Freshmen	+ .098 Position	NS
Sophomores	+ .123 Position	NS
Juniors	+ .091 Position	NS
Seniors	+ .275 Position	< .05

and evaluation strategies we utilize, (3) the types of teacher-student relations we foster, and (4) the general climate in which teaching and learning take place. In the remainder of this chapter, I will briefly explore each of these strategies.

Curriculum Design. Nursing curricula should gradually introduce students to conflict, provide independent study experiences, and offer increasingly complex courses in a variety of disciplines. (In other words, students should not be allowed to take nothing but 100-level courses.) They should participate in planned experiences with students from other disciplines so that they can be exposed to others' ways of thinking and reasoning, and they should be introduced to their major in their freshman year (to give the faculty time to enhance their development as fully as possible and to take advantage of the well-known flexibility and openness of freshmen).

We must explain to students that nursing is an imperfect discipline, that uncertainty and ambiguity are integral to our practice, and that the real world contains problems that cannot be solved, despite the best efforts of the best educated. And then we must allow them to say, "I don't know," and work with them to reach reasonable solutions to problems. We should place them first in situations where there is a large margin for error. This might help keep them from acquiring, as they often seem to, such an overwhelming fear of killing someone that they never take a risk or act independently. In addition, we should reconsider the wisdom of placing students first in wellness centers with healthy individuals. Health is an extremely complex concept, and a wellness center is a much less controlled and predictable setting than a hospital.

Teaching and Evaluation Strategies. The learner characteristics implied by various positions on Perry's continuum (Table 5) should be

Table 5

Position	Sources of Support	Sources of Challenge	Primary Intellectual Tasks	Evaluation Issues	View of Peers, Learning Process	View of the Role of the Student	View of the Role of the Instructor	View of Knowledge
2: Dualish	High degree of structure. Concrete examples. Careful sequencing, timing of diversity. Environment where people are treated kindly. Modeling on part of instructor. Chance to practice skills.	Ambiguity, multiple perspectives, uncertainty—especially by an authority; any disagreement between two respected authorities; concept of independent thought.	Learning basic information, definitions of words, concepts, and to identify parts of the whole. Beginning to compare and contrast things.	Evaluation directly related to sense of self. Bad/wrong answer = bad/wrong person. Real concern if teacher, content, and/or evaluation format is fuzzy.	Peers are not a legitimate source of knowledge or learning.	Role is to receive the information or knowledge and to demonstrate having learned the right answers.	Source of knowledge. Role is to give the knowledge to student. Good instructor equals absolute authority and knower of truth.	All knowledge is known. There is a certainty that right and wrong answers exist for everything. Knowledge is collection of information.
3: Early Multiplicity	Clarity of evaluation procedures and assignment instructions. Peers are big source of support. Comfort that we know the right process and that the right answer is out there.	Complexity—initially seen as quantity, not quality. Evaluation causes great concern. Learning processes as opposed to facts. Trying to determine which of the multiples is really right.	Can do compare and contrast tasks. Can see multiples—perspectives, parts, opinions, evaluations, difference between process and content. Use supportive evidence.	Evaluation is the primary issue. Often related to amount of time, work, "style," and quantity focus. Fairness is a major issue in judging, assignments, amount of work.	Peers are now more legitimate. Value views of peers, but still see the Instructor as the final authority.	Role is to learn how to learn, how to do the processes called for, to apply oneself, and to work hard.	Source of right way to find knowledge, of how to learn. Role is to model "the way" or process.	Most knowledge is known. All is knowable (first view of learning as a *process* that students can learn). Certainty that there exists a right way to find right answers. Realize that some areas of knowledge are "fuzzy."

4: Late Multiplicity	Enjoy diversity. Tend to balk at structure. Seek independence. Comfort with different formats, although may clearly prefer one. Can play the intellectual "game" fairly well.	Demand to use evidence to support opinion. Accepting responsibility in learning. For some, learning to listen to authority again. For others, learning to think independently.	Good at analysis. Can do some synthesis. Critique with positives and negatives. Use supportive evidence well. Relate learning to other issues. Learn to think in abstractions.	"New truth"—independent thought should get good grades. Are learning to accept qualitative criteria as legitimate in evaluation.	Peers' opinions are legitimate, but may not be listened to. One's opinion is just as good/bad as everyone else's.	Role is to learn to think for oneself and to use supportive evidence. Independence of thought is valued.	Source of the process of thinking—modeling the use of supportive evidence—modeling "the way they want us to think." Instructor can also be completely discounted.	While in some areas we have certainty about knowledge, in most we don't know for sure. Certainty that there is no certainty. Hence, "do your own thing"—one opinion's as valid as all others.
5: Contextual Relativism	Feel comfortable moving across contexts—have the intellectual tools to do so. Feeling of intellectual mastery. Comfortable seeking aid of appropriate authority/expert.	Requirement of choice or commitment. How to choose between equally good alternatives. Highly challenged to intellectual excellence.	Relate learning in one context to another. Look for relationships. See complexity. Can evaluate, conclude, support own analysis. Can synthesize. Can adapt, modify, and expand concepts.	Evaluation of work can be separated from evaluation of self. Understand that a good critique has positives and negatives. See evaluation as legitimate process/part of learning.	Peers are legitimate sources of learning if they use contextual presentation of perspectives.	Role is to use intellect, to shift from context to context, and to apply rules of adequacy to information.	Source of expertise. Role of expert/guide/consultant within the framework of "rules of adequacy" and within context. One earns authority through having expertise.	All knowledge is contextual. All knowledge is disconnected from "absolute truth." Right and wrong, adequate and inadequate, can exist within a specific context and are judged by "rules of adequacy."

*Adapted from Cornfeld, J.L. & Knefelkamp, L.L. (1979).

taken into account in the selection of teaching and evaluation strategies. We must curb our fondness for lecturing and instead use our classroom interactions with students to encourage students to process information rather than merely collect it. To this end, we should increase our use of role-playing, debate, discussion, the Socratic method, and the art of questioning.

In addition, we should assign readings in which different authors have different positions or come to different conclusions, rather than rely on a single textbook all the time; constant use of one textbook conveys to students the notion that there is one and only one right way to think and reason and do things. We should employ objective-type tests sparingly, since paper-and-pencil tests reinforce an emphasis on right answers, concreteness, and facts, at the expense of process. We should, instead, use essay exams, position papers, action projects, logs or journals, and reaction papers as means to evaluate learning.

Students might also benefit from increased use of formative evaluation, in which we encourage them to experiment and give them feedback on actions or ideas as they develop. By allowing students to choose the topics they will study, or perhaps even the assignments they will complete in a course, we will enhance their cognitive development. We limit our students' development when we emphasize such petty concerns as the exact number of pages for an assignment, the exact number of articles and texts to be cited in a bibliography, or the precise size of the margins in a paper.

On the whole, dualistic students prefer a high degree of structure, a limited amount of diversity, a great deal of personal interaction with the teacher, and concrete learning. Relativistic students, on the other hand, prefer a low degree of structure, a large amount of diversity, a moderate amount of personal interaction with the teacher, and vicarious learning. When selecting teaching and evaluation strategies, we should take care to provide some experiences that will support the students' level of cognitive development (i.e., to offer or use those strategies they prefer) and to balance these with some experience that will challenge them (i.e., to offer or use those strategies they do not prefer). In this way, we will enhance their cognitive development.

Teacher-Student Relationships. Students' cognitive development is enhanced when their relationships with their teachers are open, honest, and balanced between challenge and support. Teachers who acknowledge their mistakes, admit when they do not know something, and think problems through with students do their students a great service by helping them to see that there is a great deal of uncertainty and ambiguity in the world and that knowing the right answer is not always possible, or even desirable.

Teachers and students should be partners in learning, not adversaries. Teachers should get to know their students' individual strengths and goals, allow them to design their own learning experiences, and give them extensive feedback. Teachers should be facilitators of learning, not dictators, and their behavior should reflect relativism and commitment in relativism rather than dualism.

Overall Climate for Learning. We can also try to redesign the overall academic climate in such a way as to enhance students' cognitive development. Involving students in faculty committees exposes them to diverse opinions and helps them to see how problems are thought through and managed. Inviting students to attend faculty forums where research is discussed allows them to see how faculty members struggle to identify a problem and study it. Providing opportunities outside the classroom for students and faculty to engage in open dialogue and offering good academic advisement programs that are sensitive to student goals can do a great deal to foster the cognitive development of nursing students.

CONCLUSIONS

We need graduates who are able to be creative and willing to take risks. Still, however, higher education

> far too often stifles the inherent creativity of the student. (Carnegie Foundation for the Advancement of Teaching, 1985, p. 22)
>
> The development of creativity in the student is discouraged by fear of censure, or distrust, or fear of failure; a stifling atmosphere; attempts to closely control behavior and thinking; restricted communications; the assumption, in the classroom and in texts, that there is one right answer to every problem; and a passive role. (p. 22)
>
> Creativity and independence of mind are encouraged when students learn to question; select projects or research topics themselves (within whatever framework is necessary); and learn how concepts are related. (p. 22)
>
> The values teachers hold, and their ability to act as role models, also seem to play an important role in producing creative students. (p. 22)

Less structured, more self-directed learning experiences—in which both competition *and* cooperation are encouraged, skepticism and inquisitiveness are approved of, freedom of choice exists, and independence in learning is permitted and even expected—foster the growth of creativity and cognitive development.

Fitzpatrick (1987) argues that

> to survive, nursing education must produce quality products. We must judge the outcomes of the educational process based on universally accepted criteria related to the characteristics of educated persons as well as to the characteristics of competent professional nurses. (p. 214)

Nurses' collective self-concept and self-esteem is at an all-time low. Our professional value system is confused, and nurse educators have contributed to that confusion.

> By abandoning our concern for developing affective behaviors in our students, we have failed to reinforce the very value system that motivates and attracts people of good character to the field. (p. 214)

To date, we have placed too little emphasis on outcomes. We have focused too much on nursing and support courses and the result is that "the occupational orientation of the curriculum overshadows a true educational thrust" (p. 215).

We need to help students learn to respond to and interact with the ideas of others, to take into account diverse ways of thinking, to accept and confront differences, and to rework their thinking to incorporate more possibilities and perspectives. We must think of these developments as educational outcomes, outcomes that are at least as important as the ones usually acknowledged.

REFERENCES

Association of American Colleges. (1985). Integrity in the college curriculum. *Chronicle of Higher Education, 29*(22), 12, 13, 18–22.

Bloom, A. (1987). *The closing of the American mind.* New York: Simon and Schuster.

Carnegie Foundation for the Advancement of Teaching. (1985). Higher education and the American resurgence. *Chronicle of Higher Education, 31*(3), 17, 20.

Collins, M. S. (1981). An investigation of the development of professional commitment in baccalaureate nursing students. Unpublished doctoral dissertation, Syracuse University, Syracuse, NY.

Cordts, G. (1977). *Process of change in developmental position.* Unpublished manuscript, Georgetown University, School of Nursing, Washington, DC.

Cornfeld, J. L., & Knefelkamp, L. L. (1979). Combining student stage and style in the design of learning environments. Paper presented at meeting of the American College Personnel Association, Los Angeles.

Fitzpatrick, M. L. (1987). Dimensions of quality in nursing education. *Nursing & Health Care, 8*(4), 213–216.

Frisch, N. A. (1987). Cognitive maturity of nursing students. *Image: The Journal of Nursing Scholarship, 19*(1), 25–27.

Kiener, M. E. (1984). An evaluative study of student nurse learning within shared and primary teaching modules. Paper presented at the Midwest Research-to-Practice Conference.

Knefelkamp, L. L. (1974). Developmental instruction: Fostering intellectual and personal growth of college students. Unpublished doctoral dissertation, University of Minnesota, Minneapolis.

Knefelkamp, L. L., & Slepitza, R. (1976). A cognitive-developmental model of career development: An adaptation of the Perry scheme. *The Counseling Psychologist, 6*, 53–58.

Kurfiss, J. (1975). Late adolescent development: A structural-epistemological perspective. Unpublished doctoral dissertation, University of Washington, Seattle.

National League for Nursing. (1987). *Educational outcomes: Assessment of quality—An annotated bibliography.* New York: National League for Nursing.

Perry, W. G. (1970). *Forms of intellectual and ethical development in the college years: A scheme.* New York: Holt, Rinehart and Winston.

Ravitch, D., & Finn, C. E. (1987). *What do our 17-year-olds know?* New York: Harper & Row.

Sakalys, J. A. (1984). Effects of an undergraduate research course on cognitive development. *Nursing Research, 33*(5), 290–295.

Schein, E. H. (1972). *Professional education: Some new directions.* New York: McGraw-Hill.

Study Group on the Conditions of Excellence in American Higher Education. (1984). Involvement in learning: Realizing the potential of American higher education. *Chronicle of Higher Education, 29*(9), 35, 43.

Touchton, J. G., Wertheimer, L. C., Cornfeld, J. L., & Harrison, K. H. (1977). Career planning and decision making: A developmental approach to the classroom. *The Counseling Psychologist, 6*, 42–47.

Valiga, T. M. (1982). Cognitive development and perceptions about nursing as a profession. Unpublished doctoral dissertation, Teachers College, Columbia University, New York.

Valiga, T. M. (1983). Cognitive development: A critical component of baccalaureate nursing education. *Image: The Journal of Nursing Scholarship, 15*, 115–119.

Watson, J. (1978). Conceptual systems of undergraduate nursing students as compared with university students at large and practicing nurses. *Nursing Research*, *27*(3), 151–155.

Widick, C. A. (1975). An evaluation of developmental instruction in a university setting. Unpublished doctoral dissertation, University of Minnesota, Minneapolis.

12

Curriculum Revolution: The Practice Mandate

Christine Tanner

Embedded in our everyday lives are world views and beliefs about the self which profoundly affect the way we live. Yet these remain largely implicit and unspoken. They can become apparent as we strive with others to interpret our spoken messages and our actions. Understanding such implicit assumptions can also be emancipatory. To that end, this paper will make explicit some of the views and assumptions which have been embedded in and have dominated our practice as nurse educators.

The first part of the paper is drawn largely from the writing of Donald Schon, an MIT social scientist who has done a thoughtful study of the practice professions and their place in higher education (Schon, 1983). This is primarily to provide some context for the second and more important part of the paper. In part 2, I will explore the way in which we have formalized the concerns of practice in our nursing curricula, focusing on longstanding assumptions about the nature of nursing practice, in general, and about the nature of clinical judgment in nursing, in particular.

THE TECHNICAL RATIONALITY MODEL OF KNOWLEDGE

Schon (1983) claims that the model of what he terms technical rationality has dominated the education of professions. In this view, professional activity consists of "instrumental problem solving made rigorous by application of scientific theory and technique" (p. 21). Practice consists of problem solving based on specialized scientific knowledge. The work of the professional is to be thoroughly familiar with knowledge which has been developed and tested through research, and then apply this knowledge to solving the problems of everyday practice. This view of practice and the relationship between knowledge and practice has powerfully shaped our thinking in nursing education.

At first it may be difficult to consider the possibility that there exists another viable point of view; that is, that professional practice should or could consist of other than rational problem solving founded on a sound scientific base. This is, after all, the dominant view of nursing practice. It shows up everywhere in the literature on the relationship between theory, practice, and research. Common views about this relationship are: (1) theory and research exist to guide our practice; (2) the best practice is research-based; and (3) there is a need for more systematic research by which to provide a scientific basis for our practice. Although many authors acknowledge that questions for research might derive from practice, the flow of knowledge is clearly from research and theory to practice. The clinician is often faulted because of his or her failure to use research in practice. As a result, large-scale projects have been mounted to promote clinicians' use of research.

Schon (1983) points out that this notion of application leads to a view of professional knowledge as a hierarchy in which general principles occupy the highest level and concrete problems occupy the lowest. According to Schein (1973), there are three components to professional knowledge: (1) an underlying discipline, or basic science component upon which practice rests or from which it is developed; (2) an applied science component from which many day-to-day diagnostic procedures and problem solutions are derived; and (3) a skills and attitudinal component concerning the actual performance of services to the client, using the underlying basic and applied knowledge.

In nursing, we order our curricula along the same lines of this hierarchy. First we study the basic sciences as foundational to the applied science of nursing. For example, we assume that we cannot study asepsis until the course in microbiology is completed. Handwashing is the skill component for our applied study of asepsis. As an aside, let me point out that this hierarchy of knowledge is paralleled in the hierarchy of nursing roles. The scientist has highly esteemed status, then educators who help apply the science, and finally the clinicians at the bottom of the hierarchy.

The assumptions embedded in our curricular practices are not unlike those of other professions. But it is time to examine the assumptions that practice is *only* rigorous problem solving when applying scientific principles, and that the important and true knowledge for practice is derived from scientific research.

Schon (1983) claims that there is a crisis in the practice disciplines because this view of knowledge for practice does not meet the reality of practice. He describes the changing character of situations in practice which limit the utility of traditional scientific knowledge as the primary route to problem resolution. He points out several characteristics of practice: complexity, instability, uncertainty, and value conflict. Let us examine these characteristics more closely as they pertain to the practice of nursing, then reflect on the potential for a usable, standardized, and generalizable knowledge base for practice.

Complexity

Our scientific knowledge specifies that, all things being equal, a certain percentage of patients will respond positively to a particular intervention. Seldom in practice are all things equal. Moreover, we seldom know the extent to which this patient is like the greater proportion of patients who responded positively to the intervention. The judgment to use a scientifically based intervention is far more complex than what is assumed by the model of technical rationality and the instrumental application of scientifically based knowledge.

Instability

Our practice is changing rapidly and the development of scientific knowledge is hardly keeping pace. Because of this, too many questions in practice remain unanswered. Even if professional knowledge were to catch up with the new demands of practice, the improvement in professional performance would be transitory. The role of the nurse will continually be reshaped over the next decades by the reorganization of health and disease care. As the role changes, so will the demand for usable knowledge.

Uncertainty

The situations of practice are not problems to be solved but are problematic situations characterized by uncertainty, ambiguity, and indeterminancy. Nurses are not confronted with problems that are independent of one another but with dynamic situations of inordinate complexity and changing, interacting problems. Schon (1983) cites Russell Ackoff, who refers to such situations as "messes." Problems are abstractions extracted from "messes" by analysis.

Value Conflicts

Practitioners are frequently embroiled in conflicts of values, goals, purposes, and interests. Nurses are faced with pressures for increased efficiency in the context of contracting budgets. Patients are sent home without an adequate system of care; the goals of the institution for containing costs may be in direct conflict with the goals of quality patient care.

In summary, the argument Schon (1983) offers is based on four aspects: (1) that practice has traditionally been viewed as the instrumental application of research-based knowledge to problem solving; (2) that our educational approaches reflect a hierarchy with practice knowledge derived from higher forms of knowledge; (3) that the higher up in the hierarchy of knowledge, the more standardized and generalizable it is; and (4) that the kinds of problems (or "messes") faced by nurses in their practice requires far greater knowledge than that which is offered by traditional science. Schon offers a serious challenge to the way in which we think about practice, and the way in which we organize our curricula as a reflection of this view. An alternative conception of knowledge and the relationship between knowledge and practice may be instructive to our deliberations about curriculum change.

OTHER VIEWS OF KNOWLEDGE AND THEIR RELATIONSHIP TO PRACTICE

The notion that there are multiple ways of knowing may now be familiar through the writings of such scholars as Munhall (1982), Oiler (1982), Carper (1978), and Benner (1983, 1984; Benner & Wrubel, 1982). Benner has brought to nursing some very important notions about knowing drawn from Polanyi and the Heideggerian view of being in the world. In Benner's study of expert nurses, she found that nurses discover ways to deal competently with the ambiguities and value conflicts of practice.

There is a knowing in practice which shows up in the spontaneous, intuitive performance of the actions of everyday life. This knowing, in Polanyi's (1958) terms, is tacit, implicit in our patterns of action and in our feel for the stuff with which we are dealing. It seems that this knowing is embedded in the practice. Every competent practitioner can recognize phenomena, a pattern associated with a way of coping, or more subtle patterns which serve as an early warning of an impending problem, for which the practitioner cannot give a reasonably accurate or complete description.

To provide an illustration of such tacit knowing, I refer to our study on intuition in clinical judgment (Benner & Tanner, 1987). We observed nurses in the intensive care unit, and interviewed them about their judgments. One nurse was caring for a young female patient who was suffering from a liver disease which sometimes affects pregnant women. The woman appeared unresponsive. In response to my opening question about the patient's status, the nurse stated:

> She's more responsive than she was yesterday, but it's not real consistent. Most of the time she'll open her eyes when you talk with her. She says she's not in any pain, but I find this hard to believe because she's had a C-section. She's got that awful tube in her mouth, and we tie her down. She's more cooperative when we go to turn her, when we tell her whether we're turning her to her left or to her right. Then she starts swinging her body a little bit, not like lifting her arm up and going for the side rail, but not as resistant as she was yesterday.

This kind of qualitative distinction is difficult to describe. Yet this nurse was unusual in her ability to provide illustrations of her judgment concerning the slighly improved health of her patient. But difficulty in describing is not a case of being inarticulate. Rather, it is an implicit knowing that has not been formalized in rational language as appropriate scientific thought. In day-to-day practice the nurse makes innumerable judgments of quality for which she cannot state adequate criteria or rules. And even when the clinician makes conscious use of research-based theories and techniques, he or she is dependent on tacit recognitions, judgments, and skillful performances.

Benner (1983), drawing on the work of Polanyi and Kuhn, has made a distinction between "knowing that" and "knowing how." "Knowing that" knowledge is the formal knowledge in the curriculum, the instrumental and theoretical knowledge that makes up the course taught in the classroom. "Knowing how," or tacit knowledge, is practical knowledge and dependent on experience. In our approach to curriculum development we have recognized as legitimate only theoretical knowing, and have largely neglected the knowledge of experience.

The possibility that the technical model of higher education for the professions may not be the most functional in terms of preparing skilled clinicians is now apparent. However, there is an alternative model which, while accepting theoretical knowledge as a necessary ingredient for learning from practice, elevates the status of practice and knowledge from practice to being the lifeblood of expert performance. There is a knowing in practice which can and must inform our curriculum planning.

FORMALIZATION OF KNOWLEDGE IN THE CURRICULUM

The curriculum is our best attempt to formalize the knowledge and skills needed for practice. It is our way to put into language the concern of practice as we understand it. By concern in practice, I mean the kinds of issues with which nurses must deal. For example, in practice, we are concerned with making the best clinical judgments possible; we must prepare nurses to make astute clinical judgments, to make accurate and relevant observations, to draw inferences from those observations, and to determine appropriate nursing actions. In our curricula, we have formalized this concern as a rational, sequential model of problem solving—the nursing process—frequently operationalized as the written nursing care plan.

In the 1960s, the formalization of the nursing process was a revolutionary development. It was an acknowledgment that nurses were thinkers, not just doers. It was the application of the scientific method applied to practice. But we must ask now in the 1980s, does this formalization capture the essence of clinical judgment?

Before I consider this question in more detail, I will provide other illustrations of this way of thinking about curriculum—that is, that curriculum is the formalization of practice concerns. Illness, of course, is another concern in practice, the lived experience of our patients in coping with their diseases, their symptoms, and their changes in life style. The formalization of illness, however, quite often is disease, with the symptom being viewed as an indicator of the disease rather than an experience which has meaning for the patient. Another concern in practice is caring, our intimate connectedness with inordinate healing power. Its formalization is empathy, therapeutic communication, advocacy, and assertiveness. This interpretation of practice concerns and their formalization may not be met with unanimous agreement, but it does provide a vehicle to think about why we have included certain kinds of content in the curriculum and in what way that material may (or may not) be related to practice.

Now formalization is not an evil. A formalization is essential to provide the novice with guideposts and rules for safe entry into professional practice. However, formalizations have some charateristics which tell us that they must frequently and carefully be scrutinized for the adequacy with which they represent practice. These characteristics include the following:

1. A formalization is a representation. It gives us a way to view a situation. But it is only one representation and there may be other perspectives. It is not absolute truth.
2. As a representation and as one view, it may miss the target.
3. Formalizations are inevitably incomplete.
4. The formalization may be so abstract that multiple meanings are possible (and even likely) and the intended meaning is lost. For example, the maxim that nursing treats the whole patient is quite abstract and there are multiple concrete interpretations of this maxim.
5. There is a profound tendency to deify our formalization as being identical to the concern. Then we lose sight of the original concern. Such is the case, I believe, with the nursing process as substitute for the practice concern of clinical judgment.

THE FORMALIZATION AND THE PRACTICE OF CLINICAL JUDGMENT

Let us now take a closer look at the concern of practice of clinical judgment and its formalization in the nursing process. In this section, I will discuss some of my own research on clinical judgment and some of the turns that it has taken as a result of my own new awareness.

As a beginning nurse educator in the early 1970s, I adopted the prevailing approach to teaching clinical judgment as the nursing process. It provided a clear step-by-step linear approach to nursing judgments, a rational model which encouraged the students to clearly identify their assessment data, their plans stated as patient-centered objectives, their nursing orders and the accompanying scientific rationale, and their evaluation of the effectiveness and efficiency of the plan. I gradually became aware of the fact that while some students could write elegant care plans, these same students lacked flexibility to respond to rapidly changing practice situations, or the practical know-how to truly do the interventions. What I was most keenly aware of was that these students had no sense of salience regarding assessment data. They would collect it, and this practice seemed to get no better with time. Moreover, they seemed to have no ability to extract any meaning from the data.

In 1975, I began to research clinical problem solving. In the 10 years that followed, in an effort to understand the underlying processes of clinical judgment, I applied a rational/cognitive model of problem solving to the study of nursing students and nurses. My implicit assumption, which I did not understand until just recently, was that clinical judgment is a rational process. The meaning of this will become clear through illustrations from the research.

Actually, there are several approaches to the study of clinical judgment within the rationalist paradigm. The typical study is directed at one of two goals: (1) to compare the performance of clinicians in deriving a decision with that prescribed by a statistical model or (2) to describe the actual thought processes used by clinicians in deriving a diagnosis or determining appropriate interventions.

As an example of the former, Grier (1976) conducted a study to determine if "intuitive" decisions by nurses were in agreement with those derived by a statistical model. The model used describes the selection of an action or set of actions based on a subjective assignment of value to probable outcomes of those actions. The use of this model requires the assignment of the likelihood of certain outcomes associated with specified actions. Each outcome also has some value assigned to it. Given these subjectively assigned probabilities and values, it is possible to derive mathematically the preferred outcome. It assumes that the human judge is an intuitive statistician, that it is preferable to quantify the probabilities and values, and that the resulting decision will be better than if these probabilities and values are left unspecified. It also assumes that we can specify all relevant attributes of the situation to feed into the model.

Grier (1976) compared the decisions made intuitively with those made by the mathematical model and found agreement nearly 60 percent of the time. She concluded that a systematic and objective process was used in making most of these decisions, resulting in a justifiable choice of action for achieving the desired goal.

In my own research, I rejected this model, since my interest was more in line with attempting to describe the actual thought processes of clinical judgment. My work, up until recently, was placed squarely on information processing theory drawn from the work of Newell and Simon (1972) in artificial intelligence. This theory describes problem-solving behavior as an interaction between an information processing system (the problem solver) and a task environment (the task, as described by the experimenter). It is assumed that human information processing capacity is limited by memory constraints, and that strategies must be used to adapt these limitations to the demands of the task environment.

The model of diagnostic reasoning advanced by Elstein, Shulman, and Sprafka (1978) describes strategies which diagnosticians use to adapt to the large amounts of information available in most diagnostic tasks. The model includes four major activities: (1) problem sensing, attending to initially available cues; (2) activating diagnostic hypotheses which may explain the initial cues presented; (3) gathering data which generally are hypothesis-directed (i.e., data are sought for ruling in, ruling out, or refining the hypothesis); and (4) evaluating the hypotheses. Elstein argued that early hypotheses serve as a "chunking" mechanism, conserving short-term memory space by clustering clinical data into familiar diagnostic patterns.

My associates and I sought to determine if this model of diagnostic reasoning described the strategies used by nurses and junior and senior nursing students (Tanner, Padrick, Westfall, & Putzier, 1987; Westfall, Tanner, Putzier, & Padrick, 1986). Subjects were presented with brief videotaped vignettes depicting a patient experiencing one or more problems. The subjects' task was to seek additional information from the examiner until they had derived the most likely diagnosis(es) and determined appropriate interventions. During their information seeking, they were instructed to "think aloud"; these verbalizations were transcribed and analyzed for the number and type of diagnostic hypotheses; the earliness with which hypotheses were activated; the number of cues sought in information gathering; the type of information-gathering approach (e.g., hypothesis testing, cue exploration); the adequacy of the information used to evaluate the diagnostic hypotheses; and the accuracy of the diagnosis. They found that all subjects activated diagnostic hypotheses early. Groups could be distinguished by only two measures: the degree to which they used systematic information gathering and the accuracy of the final diagnosis.

Several other studies on clinical judgment in nursing have been conducted within the rationalist perspective. Hammond, Kelly, Schneider, and Vancini (1967) conducted the only other study comparing nursing performance with a statistical model. Corcoran (1986a; 1986b) used information processing theory to study the processes used by expert and novice hospice nurses in making decisions regarding administration of pain medications. Other investigators (Gordon, 1980; Cianfrani, 1984; Matthews & Gaul, 1979) have used concept attainment theory as a framework for research on processes of nursing diagnosis.

A singular perception emerges from these studies within the rationalist perspective: the nursing process does not capture the dynamic interactive thinking processes of diagnosis or planning. The process clearly is not as linear as we might think. Those of us involved in this area of research are now questioning the extent to which the written nursing care plan, as the primary instructional method, is likely to be helpful to nursing students in learning this dynamic process (Tanner, 1987; Corcoran, 1986a).

Along with this insight from the research, the rational model also did not seem to capture some of the more important aspects of clinical judgment. There were numerous unexplained phenomena, such as the ability to zero in on the right region for assessment, the ability to recognize which data are important to attend to and which can be ignored, the ability to recognize a pattern and act on that recognition without consciously labeling it, and the important role of emotion in clinical judgment.

In contrast, the rational model (as emphasized in nursing process, information processing theory, decision theory, and the model of technical rationality previously described) all assume that action is the result of rational and logical procedures mediated by cognitive processes. When these are not obvious or do not show themselves in the protocols of experts, it is that the processes are too rapid to access. In other words, they are unconscious. The rational model also assumes it is possible to make explicit and to formalize the knowledge used by the clinician in making judgments.

About the time that these concerns regarding the research model were rising, Benner (1984) published her early work on the development of expertise in nursing. Her work, as well as that of others (Pyles & Stern, 1983; Phillips & Rempusheski, 1985), provides a stark contrast to the rationalist models. Benner's initial work, as well as subsequent research on the role of intuition in clinical judgment (Benner & Tanner, 1987), uses hermeneutic inquiry, based on Heideggerian phenomenology.

Hermeneutic Inquiry

The object of study in hermeneutic inquiry is the semantic or textual structure of everyday practical activity, what people actually do when they are engaged in the practical tasks of life. Heidegger (1962) distinguished three modes of engagement that people have with their surroundings. The *practical* mode is the most basic. This is the mode of practical day-to-day activities, in which one's awareness is essentially holistic; that is, persons' awareness of the situation in which they are engaged is not as an arrangement of discrete physical objects, but as a network of interrelated projects. The *reflective* mode is entered when the individual encounters some problem in practical activity. The source of the breakdown of action becomes salient in a way it was not in the ready-to-hand mode. The source of the breakdown is still seen as an aspect of the task, rather than as a context-free object. The *theoretic* mode is entered only when the individual detaches him or herself from ongoing practical activity and relies on the use of rational, logical processes to deal with the breakdown.

In this view, the practical mode characterizes expert clinical judgment. The expert's perspective of a patient situation is holistic, not broken down into discrete elements. This is contrary to the rationalist assumption that expert clinical judgment is characterized by detached theorizing and analytic logical processes.

The *practical* mode also is the starting place for hermeneutic inquiry. The study of clinical judgment using hermeneutics is the study of what nurses actually do when they are engaged in the practical tasks of delivering nursing care. The hermeneutic approach seeks to make explicit the practical understanding of human actions through their interpretation.

In her study of skill acquisition, Benner (1984) interviewed and observed experienced nurses, newly graduated nurses, and senior nursing students, as well as pairs of newly licensed nurses and their more experienced nurse preceptors. During the interviews, nurses were asked to describe situations which stood out for them. Using the interview and observation data for textual interpretation, Benner provided evidence that expert judgment derives from a grasp of the whole situation—a qualitative or perceptual assessment based on a combination of "the senses of touch, smell and sight and on the interpretation of a patient's physical, verbal and behavioral expression" (Benner & Wrubel, 1982, p. 12). These holistic judgments differed from the objective, measurable judgments such as those described in the rationalist models. In a study using grounded theory strategies, Pyles and Stern (1983) identified the formation of a "gestalt" or achievement of insight about a patient situation, similar to Benner's description.

In subsequent research on clinical judgment within this perspective, Benner and Tanner (1987) described aspects of intuition. Drawing on the work of Dreyfus and Dreyfus (1986), they defined intuition as "understanding without a rationale" and not a "mystical or accidental human capacity" (p. 29). In their pilot study, expert nurses were interviewed and observed in their practice. The narrative accounts provided by the nurses contain rich descriptions of expert clinical judgment.

Several aspects of intuition described in this study are relevant to this discussion.

1. *Pattern recognition* is the perceptual ability that enables human beings to recognize configurations and relationships without analytically specifying the components of the patterns. A good example of this ability is face recognition; people do not analyze an individual's facial features, yet they are able to recognize people they have met by a memory of the overall facial "pattern." Patients present patterns that expert nurses learn to attend to. In contrast to this view of pattern recognition, rationalist models of clinical judgment treat pattern recognition either as a feature detection system, in which a list of features held in memory is matched against the features presented by the patient, or as a template matching scheme.
2. *Sense of salience* is the perception of things as being more or less important. The expert nurse, who has a sense of salience, will not consider all observations as pertinent; only some will stand out. Skilled observations of the patient over a long period of time allow the nurse to understand what is salient for *this* situation. A routine assessment checklist will not be as effective in situations that require highly individualized observations, such as the subtle changes occurring in head-injured patients.

Now let us examine contrasting assumptions. In this view, action precedes analytic thought rather than occurring as a result of it. The knowing is in the doing, and we may theorize about it later. There are no formal strategies of clinical judgment that can be described free of the context in which the action occurs. Rather, an understanding of any human activity must be historically and contextually situated. The knowledge used as the basis for clinical judgment is practical, derived from experience with similar and dissimilar situations. The knowledge is embedded in the practice and may or may not be rendered explicit or formal. Rational, analytic approaches to clinical judgment are characteristic of beginner rather than expert performance.

What may we conclude from this regarding the formalization of clinical judgment as nursing process? It is a formalization which is ill-suited to expertise in practice. At best, it may serve as an introductory framework which may quickly be abandoned as students gain some experience in their clinical work. It may also represent, somewhat inadequately, aspects of clinical judgment, but it cannot be considered the same as the processes of clinical judgment.

In my work with Benner, I had the opportunity to watch and talk with some of the best nurses I have ever seen. Their expertise in clinical judgment, their understanding of the lived experience of illness, their attitudes toward caring escaped the formalisms we currently use in our nursing programs. Finally, I would like to share with you an incredibly poignant paradigm case that captures the essence of this expertise and, at the same time, the limits of formalism.

This paradigm case was presented by a skilled coronary care unit nurse during a group interview. The man she is discussing was in the coronary care unit for cardiomyopathy.

> We had a young man, 22 years old, who I will never forget. He was about 2 and 1/2 hours from home, and up here by himself. I think he knew that he was very ill but he didn't really understand how ill. He didn't understand that he was actually terminal. The impression I had was that it was important for us as a nursing staff to know him as a person and to care for him. And he was very personable. I took care of him three days in a row for 12-hour shifts. I admitted him and chose to stay with him. He was very hopeful that something would be found, that he would feel better. Sometimes he would even say: "Oh, I don't feel too bad now." But his readings would be just about the same and really he didn't have an improvement. So he was really searching, I think, and it made my heart go out to him.
>
> He made a point to share a lot of personal aspects of his life. And not everybody does that. [I: Give me an example of the kinds of things he shared.] What he liked to do with his free time, how he met his fiance, how he never thought he would be in a hospital being so young, how he couldn't wait to go home because he had these things he planned to do, and the wedding was in 6 months and gee, he had never even been to a wedding before and now he was going to have his own. He told me what his fiance did for a living, and how he hoped to go into business with his father. Things like that, little things but he seemed to want to talk about his life al-

most every time I went into his room. I don't know, maybe he did realize how sick he was.

[I: How did you respond to that?] It made me sad, but I was flattered that he wanted to talk to me. I just listened and would say, "Is that right?" or "How nice that you met this person." I didn't ask him, I wanted to let him say what he wanted to say.

They made the decision not to intubate him, even though it is a very hard decision to make, and you feel very ambivalent. He became very breathless. Now the point was just to make him as comfortable as possible. He felt more comfortable in the chair. So he sat in the chair. He wanted a popsicle. He got a popsicle. He wanted to drink some water. Fine, he could have water if he wanted it. We started giving him small doses of morphine to see if that would help with his anxiety. Medically, they didn't want to give more potent respiratory depressants like valium because they felt that that might harm him. However, in retrospect, I wish they could have calmed him somewhat. But it has given me tremendous empathy for people who are short of breath. It's an awful way to go because he was conscious to the very end. He also kept pulling me back. Anytime I tried to leave the room he would grab my arm and say: "Don't leave me. Don't leave me." So I stayed with him and had someone else take over my other patient assignments.

I held his hand, I rubbed his neck. We brought a radio into the room so he could listen to rock and roll. Little things like that. He wanted a fan. We located a fan on another floor. These little comfort measures. I think he was very afraid of dying alone, and even though I was just his nurse, it meant something to him.

If we were to try to formalize this paradigm case in abstractions describing the nurse-patient relationship or the processes of the nurse's clinical judgments, the important meaning would be, in large measure, lost. While our efforts to formalize the process of nursing care are important to the educational endeavor, we must avoid our tendency to equate them with the concern(s) of practice which we are trying to represent.

We have much to learn from practice and from experts in practice. Now when I think of curriculum revolution, I do not think of developing more elegant and detailed formal models to be passed on to the next generation of nurses, for them to take and apply in their practice. Rather, I am struggling with ways in which the concerns of practice can truly be addressed by our educational activities, where classroom learning might be the application of practice rather than the other way around. I hope that you will join me in this struggle.

REFERENCES

Benner, P. (1984). *From novice to expert: Power and excellence in nursing practice.* Palo Alto, CA: Addison-Wesley.

Benner, P. (1983). Uncovering the knowledge embedded in clinical practice. *Image: The Journal of Nursing Scholarship, 15*(2), 36–41.

Benner, P., & Tanner, C. (1987). Clinical judgment: How expert nurses use intuition. *American Journal of Nursing, 87,* 23–31.

Benner, P., & Wrubel, J. (1982). Skilled clinical knowledge: The value of perceptual awareness. *Nurse Educator, 7*(3), 11–17.

Carper, B. A. (1978). Fundamental patterns of knowing in nursing. *Advances in Nursing Science, 1*(1), 13–23.

Cianfrani, K. L. (1984). The influence of amounts and relevance of data on identifying health problems. In M. J. Kim, G. K. McFarland, & A. M. McLane (Eds.), *Classification of nursing diagnoses: Proceedings of the fifth national conference.* St. Louis: C.V. Mosby, pp. 159–161.

Corcoran, S. (1986a). Task complexity and nursing expertise as factors in decision making. *Nursing Research, 35,* 107–112.

Corcoran, S. (1986b). Planning by expert and novice nurses in cases of varying complexity. *Research in Nursing and Health, 9,* 155–162.

Dreyfus, H. L. (1979). *What computers can't do: The limits of artificial intelligence.* New York: Harper & Row.

Dreyfus, H. L., & Dreyfus, S. E. (1986). *Mind over machine.* New York: The Free Press.

Elstein, A., Shulman, L., & Sprafka, S. (1978). *Medical problem solving.* Cambridge, MA: MIT Press.

Gordon, M. (1980). Predictive strategies in diagnostic tasks. *Nursing Research, 29,* 39–45.

Grier, M. (1976). Decision making about patient care. *Nursing Research, 25*(2), 105–110.

Hammond, K. R., Kelly, K. J., Schneider, R. J., & Vancini, M. (1967). Clinical inference in nursing: Revising judgments. *Nursing Research, 16,* 38–45.

Heidegger, M. (1962). *Being and time.* (J. Macquarrie & E. Robinson, Trans.). New York: Harper & Row.

Matthews, C. A., & Gaul, A. L. (1979). Nursing diagnosis from the perspective of concept attainment. *Advances in Nursing Science, 2,* 17–26.

Munhall, P. L. (1982). Nursing philosophy and nursing science: In apposition or opposition. *Nursing Research, 31,* 176–177, 181.

Newell, A., & Simon, H. (1972). *Human problem solving.* Englewood Cliffs, NJ: Prentice-Hall.

Oiler, C. (1982). The phenomenological approach in nursing research. *Nursing Research, 31,* 178–181.

Phillips, L. R., & Rempusheski, V. F. (1985). Diagnosing and intervening for elder abuse and neglect: An empirically generated decision-making model. *Nursing Research, 34*, 134–139.

Polanyi, M. (1958). *Personal knowledge*. Chicago: University of Chicago Press.

Pyles, S. H., & Stern, P. N. (1983). Discovery of nursing gestalt in critical care nursing: The importance of the gray gorilla syndrome. *Image: The Journal of Nursing Scholarship, 15*(2), 51–57.

Schein, E. (1973). *Professional education*. New York: McGraw-Hill.

Schon, D. A. (1983). *The reflective practitioner*. New York: Basic Books.

Tanner, C. A. (1987). Teaching Clinical Judgment. In J. J. Fitzpatrick & R. L. Tauton (Eds.), *Annual review of nursing research, vol. 5*. New York: Springer, pp. 153–173.

Tanner, C. A., Padrick, K. P., Westfall, U. E., & Putzier, D. J. (1987). Diagnostic reasoning strategies of nurses and nursing students. *Nursing Research, 36*(6), 358–363.

Westfall, U. E., Tanner, C. A., Putzier, D. J., & Padrick, K. P. (1986). Clinical inference in nursing: A preliminary analysis of cognitive strategies. *Research in Nursing and Health, 9*, 269–277.

13

Curriculum Revolution: A Social Mandate for Change

Patricia L. Munhall

Like many of you here this morning, I agree to almost anything if it is three months away from the date of the request. When I was asked to speak at this NLN Nurse Educator Conference, I felt privileged and did not give the title of the paper, which was assigned by the conference planning committee, my full attention at that time. Now, three months later, if I say I won't comment on the word "mandate," I have already done so. And not to say anything further might be seen as tacit agreement to the use of sexist language, a subject particularly important in any discussion on curriculum revolution. Since this paper attends to our consciousness specifically, perhaps I should gender balance the idea of "mandate" to "humandate for change," thereby enhancing its focus.

The date of being asked to present this paper aside, its title still interests me. It reads as though a curriculum revolution is in progress and is creating, on its own, a humandate for change. Traditionally, however, this situation has been the reverse; social forces usually stimulate curriculum change. This might not be problematic if it were not for the fact that curriculum change is a slow process, generally lagging behind contemporary reality in some subjects by as much as ten years. Fahey (1987) has commented that changing a curriculum is something like moving a cemetery. I like that analogy and am reminded of cemeteries that are built upward, where one dead soul is piled up on another and another, ad infinitum, like vertical strands.

However humorous this analogy might appear, I do believe that a curriculum revolution in nursing is beginning. That we are here together this week to contemplate and explore the meaning of this beginning is itself a sufficient cause for hope. Who is to know if the fluttering of one's butterfly wings is not the beginning of a hurricane two hundred years later?

In this paper, I will examine the meanings of and the possibilities for an evolving curriculum revolution. Historically, we have used the rational model for analysis when struggling for curriculum change. We ask questions such as those before us today: what are the major trends influencing social behavior, what is the changing role of consumers, and how will all this impact on curriculum designs?

We use demographics, futurists' reports, cost constraint plans, and other important variables as well. For example, we use Naisbitt's (1982, 1984) *Megatrends*, and while they are critical of contemporary planning in general, there are always the unforseeable events that influence our daily lives to as great an extent and which are more rarely examined. We must remember that trends are trends, nothing more; they come and go. Perhaps we need to look at more enduring things. Perhaps we need to turn our discussion towards our interior selves, focusing on the ways in which we internalize social trends and individual experiences as sources of knowledge. Today, concomitant with the rational model for analysis is a growing, perhaps even "mega" acknowledgment of a potential for other ways of knowing. Often associated with women's ways is another perspective of reality where emotion, intuition, and imagination are becoming more valued.

In this spirit, I will focus on our interior perspectives, our consciousness, our perceptions, and what we mean by being human today. Therefore, while we acknowledge movement from an industrial to an imformation society, from a national to a world economy, from centralization to decentralization, and from short- to long-term orientations, let us tentatively examine less external influences; let us attend to the life in ourselves.

No doubt I will only summarily touch upon ideas of expanded consciousness, transformation as revolution, narcissism as a defense against powerlessness, nurses as an oppressed group, horizontal violence, Big Brother, retreat from freedom, retreat from thoughtfulness, the acknowledgment of values in science, shifting metaphors, and revolutionary flutterings. However, I will conclude each section with applicable thoughts for curriculum change based on interior themes as they interact with external trends.

But these are only a few of the brush strokes necessary to complete the unfinished canvas that speaks to our mutual humandate for change.

TRANSFORMATION AS REVOLUTION

It is always of interest to me how an intense scrutiny of the words we use often enables us to sidestep and avoid confronting the issue at hand. While I alluded to the examination of sexist language as part of a curriculum revolution (actually an examination of gender biasing in curriculum would be more encompassing), here I am speaking about the word *revolution*. That this word can be most anxiety-provoking should not detain us. This anxiety is appropriate, even cautionary, when faced with the task before us. Revolutionaries, however, have always placed their causes above their anxiety. Be that as it may, let us attend to the origin of that anxiety. The reality of an actual curriculum revolution in nursing education is a project that would demand from us a commitment not unlike any other revolution in thought and education. And we know the enormity of dedication, sacrifices, labor, and even bloodshed that accompany such efforts.

Bloodshed in a curriculum revolution? This is not as far-fetched as it might seem. When equated with professional lives and future careers, it is clear that many professional lives have been wounded in the quest for change. That we know this and sometimes fear it is itself a particularly forceful obstacle for those who visualize change. Yet a curriculum revolution in nursing education has begun; we are all here to discuss it, to examine it, to plan it. Indeed everyone here today might be a revolutionary at heart—a wonderful thought!

I use the word *revolution* specifically in regard to transformation. This transformation has to do with shifts in paradigm and with an expansion of consciousness. A curriculum revolution would entail both, of course: there would be a new way of thinking and a new scheme for understanding and explaining certain aspects of reality. The Women's Revolution offers a perfect example (and can serve as a prototype) of such shifts and expansion. At one time, and not so long ago, it was firmly believed that women's ovaries shrank in direct proportion to their intake of knowledge, that their brains were smaller and weighed less than a man's brains, and that they were therefore intellectually deficient. These beliefs were part of a larger paradigm of power, a paradigm that encompassed both economic and political aspects. In 1920, women could not vote, to say nothing of their wage scale in relation to mens'. In 1984, a woman ran for vice president and the business community is more responsive to wage scale parity. There is a new knowing, a new world view, a different perception; our eyes have widened, we are taking more in, and we are indeed raising consciousness.

Today, we have our own revolutionaries in nursing education. Actually, we always have or we would not be here today. We would still be dependent, docile, and respectful handmaidens, not to patients so much as to the paternal autocracy that governs our health care and educational systems. These revolutionaries are stirring the air with their questions and their criticisms, their wings are fluttering, and they seem to be part of what Ferguson (1980) calls *The Aquarian Conspiracy*. As Ferguson offers it, the conspiracy was named in response to what she found already existing around her. It was, she wrote, "The Movement That Has No Name." Describing this movement, Ferguson stated:

> The spirit of our age is fraught with paradox. It is at the same time pragmatic and transcendental. It values both enlightenment and mystery, power and humility, interdependence and individuality . . . It is short on manifestos. It seems to speak to something very old. And perhaps, by integrating magic and science, art and technology, it will succeed where all the king's horses and all the king's men failed. (p. 18)

But what exactly is the Aquarian Conspiracy? Literally, "conspire" means to breathe together; "Aquarian," love and light. The once popular song "The Age of Aquarius" celebrates the hope for a true liberation of the mind. Because we are here today, we also possess this hope. Yet movements such as this, movements animated by such a hope, are seen to attract a pejorative "unstable" element. Perhaps it is more pejorative to be "stable" in the face of social changes that demand a conscientious response. Revolutionary ideas, revolutionaries themselves, in whatever context, are often scorned and ridiculed: this we know. But the depth of courage and commitment, the visions of a better world that have led to successful revolutions: this we also know. It is something we must get to know even more.

On this program I believe we have some, though by no means all, of nursing's revolutionaries. Among the presenters we have Jean Watson, who has founded and promoted a Center for Human Caring; Christine Tanner, who has crystallized the legitimacy of intuition as a way of knowing; and Patricia Moccia, who has equated caring with social activism. We have Carolyn Oiler Boyd, who has called our attention to the philosophy of phenomenology; Nancy Diekelmann, who has challenged us on our acceptance of the Tyler model for curriculum design; Pamela Maraldo, who has stirred us up politically for humanistic reasons; and Nancy Greenleaf, who has raised our consciousness about women's work and nursing. There are others we are fortunate to hear this week, others similarly described and committed that I would place in the movement that has no name: Lucille Joel, Hans Mauch, Alma Wooley, Susan Costello, Sheila Corcoran, Carol Lindeman, Theresa Valiga, Franklin Shaeffer, Mila Aroskar, and Em Olivia Bevis.

This particular group of individuals are gathered together to promote a more humanistic society. Because we know that our curricula and the way its content is taught has everything to do with the delivery of health care, we also share an "Aquarian" aim: to breathe new life into the process of nursing education in response not to the breakdown but hopefully to a breakthrough in advancing the human community.

But we move tentatively, both as nurses and, for the most part, as women. Perhaps we need to be bolder. Perhaps we need to expand our consciousness further, and in that expansion open doors, the front to let fresh air in and the back to let stale air out. Perhaps the old ideas and assumptions concerning nursing curricula and the delivery of health care do not fit anymore. Perhaps they are paradigms that inhibit our growth rather than spur it onward and should be abandoned.

Implications of this act are profound and require, as we move forward, a new paradigm. General aspects of this paradigm are presented in Table 1.

Table 1
Implications for Curriculum Within the Theme of the Aquarian Conspiracy

Suggested processes:	People movement Projects for: loneliness, hunger, the homeless, alienation, ethical and moral problems, ecology, poverty	Fostering community Search for meaning Self-discovery Freedom Choices Relationships
Concrete bottom line:	Welcome the unstable. Listen to those with ideas out of the mainstream. Try to be less critical of the unknown.	

ORWELL AND HUXLEY REVISITED

The Aquarian Conspiracy is decidedly *hopeful* and is based on a deeply felt enthusiasm for things humane. While a curriculum revolution in nursing education would be congruent with this hope, one can argue that it is merely utopian. What, then, are other perspectives of our human condition that need our attention as we attempt to comprehend the nature of our world and its apparent contradictions?

Postman (1985), in what I would call a "dire warning" book entitled *Amusing Ourselves to Death,* calls to our attention the prophesies of Orwell's *1984* and Huxley's *Brave New World.* Postman's analysis focuses on the critical importance of using such prophesies to understand ourselves and our world today. For a curriculum revolution, Orwell's and Huxley's prophesies are important to ponder.

According to Postman (1985), Orwell warned us that we would be overcome by an externally imposed oppression. Big Brother would hold us prisoners in a capricious world where truth and culture are concealed. In Huxley's *Brave New World,* no Big Brother is needed to deprive people of their autonomy, maturity, and history. Huxley believed that individuals would find comfort in their oppression, adore their technologies, and that a sea of irrelevance would smother the truth. In contrasting these prophecies, Postman describes this difference: Orwell feared governmental forces that would ban books; Huxley feared that there would be no reason to ban books because there would not be an audience interested enough to read them. Huxley feared we would become a trivial culture, a culture of distractions where Big Brother does not watch us so much as we *watch* him. Postman believes that Big Brother functions today in the guise of the mass media, which is transforming the world by amusing us "to death."

"Reach out and Elect Someone" is a chapter in Postman (1985) that increases our understanding of Huxley's warning. Currently we have the 30-second political commercial where presidential candidates deliver their messages in slots between football quarters. Perhaps we should take heed of the influence of what Postman calls *media as epistemology,* a term he uses to describe how we have come to learn about our world in these last decades of the 20th century. The following example from political history contrasts this situation with one from the last century.

In the Lincoln-Douglas debates in 1858, Douglas would speak first for one hour, then Lincoln would take an hour and a half to reply, and Douglas a half hour to rebut Lincoln's response. Actually this was much shorter than usual for that time. This past November, in a televised political debate between the 1988 candidates of both the Democratic and Republican parties, which, by the way, was organized on the lines of the game show "Family Feud," each candidate had one minute to sum up his foreign policy position, the others 30 seconds to respond. Major issues were addressed in this fashion: one-minute position statements, 30-second responses. If this wasn't so frightening, it would be comical.

Why is this important in a discussion about curriculum? This is the culture in which we—faculty, students, and consumers—live. The media addresses us in snapshots, slogans, and superficial analyses geared to short attention spans. On the subject of attention spans, William Safire, the noted columnist for the New York Times, was heard to say:

> We sophisticates can listen to a speech for a half hour, but after ten minutes the average guy wants a beer.

To add to this, the other day I overheard a graduate student say with some incredulity that it took her 11 hours to do a paper. I suggest that this should only come as a surprise for the brevity of the time, not for the perceived enormity. However, this is what Postman and Huxley warn us about. We have the one-minute everything: the one-minute manager, the one-minute parent, and the one-minute statement of foreign policy. H.G. Wells (Postman, 1987) said that we are in a race between education and disaster. That race, I believe, also contains within it the seed of a social humandate for curriculum revolution. In *Brave New World*, Huxley did not find fault with people laughing but with the fact that they did not know what they were laughing about and why they stopped thinking.

Implications for a curriculum revolution within the themes discussed by Orwell and Huxley are presented in Table 2.

NARCISSISTIC INFLUENCES

Concomitant with the influence of mass media, what are other variables within our society that should be considered in curriculum planning? Lasch (1979) writes of American life in an age of diminishing expectations. While Ferguson (1980) writes of human connectedness, Lasch writes of human disconnectedness. In his book *The Culture of Narcissism*, Lasch helps us to understand why many nurse faculty, nurs-

Table 2
Implications for Curriculum Within the Orwell-Huxley Themes

Suggested processes:	Reflect on how oppression is maintained through mass media.
	Focus on critical thinking, and cognitive and moral development.
	Students must learn to speak, discuss, and debate.
	Teach more thoughtful inductive and deductive writing.
	Analyze the media's coverage of life styles, health, politics, and nursing.
Concrete bottom line:	Return to the printed word rather than adopt technological substitutes.
	Examine the trivial distractions in our society for meaning.
	Examine how students write their biographies and the biographies of others.

ing students, and consumers are unable to comprehend reality in an optimistic, transforming way. They no longer believe in the leadership of this country or its organizations. They are disillusioned, disappointed, and have turned to themselves for consolation. They have become part of the "me" generation. In effect, they no longer trust grander schemes.

Lasch (1979) posits that narcissism is a metaphor of the human condition. This idea may help us to understand the cause of a more obvious apathy or disinterest in many individuals toward societal problems. Because some people are disillusioned with grander schemes, they live for the moment, for themselves, and not for their predecessors or posterity. Because individuals believe that society is on the brink of annihilation and has no future, it makes sense to live only for the moment, to focus on private performance, and to cultivate self-attention. As a cultural phenomenon, the world view that emerges from such beliefs centers solely on the self, the sole good being individual survival. Underlying this, Lasch theorizes, is a loss of self-esteem and a self-directed rage in the face of an evident powerlessness to change this.

Such feelings can lead into the dynamics of oppressed group behavior. The narcissistic individual sees him or herself as powerless, in this case, against society. Similarly, an oppressed group sees itself as powerless against an oppressor. In nursing, this has also led to rage. As

Table 3
Implications for Curriculum Within the Theme of Narcissism

Suggested processes:	Curriculum must promote self-esteem, feeling of power, independence, cooperation, seeing and caring about the big picture, women's studies, psychology of oppressed groups, and active social participation.
Concrete bottom line:	Give up horizontal violence. Focus on the achievements of nurses and others. Accomplish social change.

Roberts (1983) points out, this rage in nursing as in other oppressed groups leads to a form of horizontal violence where we confront and vie with one another instead of the oppressor. This "submissive-aggressive" syndrome, as it is termed by Roberts, has characterized many nursing encounters when the goal has been change.

Before a curriculum revolution is possible, these feelings of powerlessness must be dealt with. Narcissistic tendencies to exclusive self-involvement and oppressed group behavior need to be analyzed. Without understanding their causes, both within the self and the world, nurses will fail to realize their curriculum revolution. Implications for curriculum within the theme of narcissism are presented in Table 3.

THE MEASUREMENT OF MAN

Another perspective advantageous to us is in recognizing weaknesses within deterministic arguments. Laudan (1977) in *Science Progress and Problems* and Gould (1981) in *The Mismeasure of Man* analyze this issue.

Laudan explicates the historicist perspective of science as process, rather than product. The process is one of human behavior and thought exhibited by practicing scientists. Rather than focusing on objectivity and the idea of a value-free science, Laudan attends to the psychological factors of individual scientists, the social forces that effect the community other than those created by scientists, the overall historical environment within which scientists work, and the non-scientific influence on scientists.

Nowhere do I believe this subjectivity is as important to recognize than in the perpetual and sometimes dangerously subtle influences of the theory of biological determinism. Gould (1981) makes this case eloquently when he states:

> We pass through this life but once. Few tragedies can be more extensive than the stunting of life, few injustices deeper than the denial of an opportunity to strive or even to hope, by a limit imposed without, but falsely identified as lying within. (p. 19)

Biological determinism is a theory of limits. It takes the current status of groups (e.g., women nurses) as a measure of where they should and must be even if it allows rare individuals the opportunity to rise because of a fortunate quirk in their biology. Biological determinism, which purports the superiority of specific races, classes, and sexes, possesses evident utility for groups in power.

I believe that it is dangerous to think that the idea of biological determinism is dead. Attribution of superiority to the male is borne out in current research studies. Attribution of superiority to white men over other races is still the norm. Even with the exceptional female present, the subsequent patriarchy is everywhere. Why is this important to a curriculum revolution? Our science is culturally embedded in a world where social prejudice still exists. As posited by Laudan (1977), historicism recognizes conscious and unconscious motivations, culture, power, and means and ends as part of the scientific enterprise. Logical positivism, with its focus on value-free science, objectivity, and quantifying proof is seriously challenged here and we have the possibility of a new philosophy of science to guide research within our curriculums. Implications for curriculum within the theme of the mismeasure of man are presented in Table 4.

SHIFTING METAPHORS

Nursing has always valued caring. In a society that refuses to value caring, however, being ordered to care raises a central dilemma for nurses (Reveby, 1987). To overcome this dilemma, the idea of caring itself is undergoing change. Gilligan (1982) has formulated a moral development model embedded in an ethic of care. The language of

Table 4
Implications for Curriculum
Within the Theme of the Mismeasure of Man

Suggested processes:	In health care and research analyze the political and cultural use of measurement. Theory of biological determinism and its effect on nursing. Social prejudice. Role theory and role expectations. The class system and health care. Injustice and inequalities: ageism, sexism, and racism. Subjective expressions of experience.
Concrete bottom line:	Introspect the extent to which we defer or play games that go along with biological determinism. Research photographs in nursing textbooks for biases. Analyze the structure of daily life. Have students write narratives and paint pictures. Take photographs of what it means to be human today.

caring, which has been confined to the private domain and largely to women, emerges now as an ethical principle grounded in the concept of social responsibility and the credo of non-violence.

Yet the idea of caring has not entirely changed within the traditional metaphoric subplot of our roles. The physician often remains as the paternal voice of authority, the nurse as the maternal figure, and the patient as the child. This role assignment of expectation may be changing but it is not absent, and the so-called patriarchal medical model is still very much with us. I believe there is also present in nursing a behaviorial metaphor based on military discipline. As educators we have diligently and with passion tried to change these models; we must not tire in this pursuit now.

I think that many of our students would recognize the scenario of the military metaphor which prizes obedience to higher ranks and subordination to orders whether from doctors or nurses. Subordination is the critical element here. Today we are attempting to change from a military metaphor to a metaphor of advocacy where our loyalty is to the patient rather than to authority. Advocacy is grounded in caring as a social responsibility and, indeed, Curtin (1979) has suggested that the concept of advocacy be seen as the philosophical basis for nursing. I am not sure whether our curricula adequately reflects this and I am not sure how many of our clients would be aware of this. Perhaps our curricula do reflect this and the settings contradict it. Whichever

Table 5
Implications for Curriculum Within Shifting Metaphors

Suggested processes:	Evaluate developmental theories. Emphasize the ethic of care. Act for patient advocacy. Develop nursing-person identity. Hear our different voices. Analyze all implications of behaviorism.
Concrete bottom line:	Protest inhumane and unsafe patient conditions. Protest whatever demeans the status of nurses. Infuse curriculum with professionalism.

is the case, in reality we practice in organ-named hospitals, on organ- or disease-named units, are sometimes called organ-named nurses, or unit-named nurses, often feeling like all we do is follow orders in military-type organizations as we try to move up the "ranks." Perhaps, because we have been socialized early on to certain values, beliefs and attitudes about the role of women, caring, and attachments, we experience many internal conflicts in this process.

Thanks to the works of individuals like Miller (1977) and Gilligan (1982), among many others, a very different perspective of women, caring, and social responsibility is making its appearance. Implications for curriculum in this shifting of dominant metaphors are presented in Table 5.

CONCLUSION

The social humandate for change calls us to conspire together in the transformation of behavioristic, externally driven curriculum to one that focuses on expanding consciousness and the subjective and intersubjective experiences of being human. Attention needs to be directed to facilitating an articulate, self-confident, self-possessed individual with social consciousness and commitment to professional ideals.

In addition to considering the external environment when planning curriculum change, we need to acknowledge our interior selves, in effect, who we are, who our students are, and who the consumer is. We need to acknowledge divergent perspectives of the human experience. We need to acknowledge that individuals choose professionalism as a way of life, most likely, while in high school and then make a career choice based on that. As part of planning curriculum change, let us also infuse nursing, both substantively and image-wise, with professionalism.

While change is characteristically slow, I do not believe we have the luxury at this time to deliberate and discuss every singular criterion for curriculum, however. We are losing women and men to more prestigious and lucrative professions. We need to compete aggressively. Our curricula must be attractive, challenging, and intellectually professional. It must also increase the status, self-esteem, and social consciousness of nursing majors.

Instead of practicing the submissive-aggressive syndrome characteristic of oppressed groups, let us take our normal energetic feelings and direct them toward changing the processes of our curricula. Less didactic, less multiple choice, less behaviorism, less militaristic characteristics, less positiveness, and more emphasis on social consciousness, social responsibility, humanism, caring, ethics, critical thinking, and the arts as well as science are necessary. So long have we worked with rational behavior styles that we must now consider the interiors, the particulars, the relational, the contextual, and the meaning of experience for both consumer and nurse.

This paper has been an attempt to hopscotch from one perspective to another in a discussion of societal influences that need our attention in curriculum planning. I have attempted to situate us in our social-cultural context and speak to interior responses that translate into external styles of behavior. I firmly believe that as our interior selves are attended to, the flutterings and stirrings about us today will lead to a curriculum revolution where change will be one of process, existentially bewildering, enchanting, and above all liberating.

REFERENCES

Curtin, L. (1979). The nurse as advocate: A philosophical foundation for nursing. *Advances in Nursing Science, 1*(3).

Fahey, E. (1987, October). *Distinguished lecture series, Teachers College, Columbia University.*

Ferguson, M. (1980). *The aquarian conspiracy.* Boston: Houghton Mifflin.

Gilligan, C. (1982). *In a different voice: Psychological theory and women's development.* Cambridge, MA: Harvard University Press.

Gould, S. (1981). *The mismeasure of man.* New York: W.W. Norton & Co.

Lasch, C. (1979). *The culture of narcissism*: New York: Warner Books.

Laudan, L. (1977). *Progress and its problems: Towards a theory of scientific growth.* Berkeley, CA: University of California Press.

Miller, J. B. (1977). *Toward a new psychology of women.* Boston: Beacon Press.

Naisbitt, J. (1982, 1984). *Megatrends.* New York: Warner Books.

Postman, N. (1985). *Amusing ourselves to death.* New York: Viking Penguin.

Reveby, S. (1987). *Ordered to care: The dilemma of American nursing 1850-1945.* New York: Cambridge University Press.

Roberts, S. J. (1983). Oppressed group behavior implications for nursing. *Advances in Nursing Science, 5*(4), 21–30.

14

Teaching Research in the Undergraduate Curriculum

Carol Lindeman

To my knowledge, nursing research has been a topic of formal study at the undergraduate level for over 25 years. For example, the programs for juniors and seniors at the University of Hawaii School of Nursing, described by Burkhalter and Kim (1976), began in 1962. At the University of Wisconsin, Eau Claire, a formal course in nursing research has been part of the curriculum since the mid-1960s. Yet it wasn't until the mid-1970s that the profession arrived at a consensus that involvement in research beginning at the baccalaureate level is essential for the advancement of the profession and its growth as a discipline.

Duffy (1987) succinctly summarizes the evolution of this consensus:

> The most important formal indication of this consensus occurred in 1972, when the Board of Directors of the National League for Nursing challenged nurse educators "to provide opportunities for students to learn to interpret research, understand its methods and significance, assess its findings, and adapt those to practice that have value." Five years later the NLN Council of Baccalaureate and Higher Degree Programs included research as one of its criteria for accreditation; and shortly thereafter, they specified this to mean that students should acquire "an understanding of the research process and its contribution to nursing practice" and have the ability "to evaluate research for the applicability of its findings to nursing actions." During the same period the American Nurses Association (ANA) Commission on Nursing Research issued a statement recom-

> mending that at the undergraduate level faculty members should introduce research early in students' education, help them to develop an attitude of inquiry, and encourage students to seek out research findings and use them in providing patient care. Although the NLN and ANA statements differed in their wording, their message was the same: baccalaureate nursing education should prepare students to be intelligent consumers of research findings and to evaluate these findings for their applicability to nursing practice. (p. 87)

In this paper, I provide an overview of the literature published between 1980 and 1987 on the what, when, and how of teaching research to undergraduate nursing students. Afterwards, I explain what I think is the major obstacle to teaching research at the undergraduate level.

THE WHAT OF TEACHING RESEARCH

Downs (1980) describes the research process as including both a theoretical aspect and a methodological aspect. In her view, the relationship of these aspects should change as the student progresses.

> At each successive level of instruction, more emphasis should be placed on theoretical considerations. At the same time, as the student attempts to solve more abstract intangible problems, the methodological component needs to become more sophisticated. At a beginning level, students can seek answers to practical problems that place minimal emphasis on the abstract connections linking question and answer. (p. 8)

Downs also urges that theory be separated from beginning research methodology.

Fleming (1980) would divide the teaching of research at the bachelor's level into five components:

1. Learning nursing. (Such knowledge is essential for helping the learner identify the problems that need study and understand basic concepts and theoretical notions.)
2. Critical and reflective thinking.
3. Problem solving. (This process should be stressed, and opportunities for identifying problems appropriate for research provided. It would be highly desirable for each learner to carry out a problem-solving project related to clinical practice or the profession of nursing.)

4. The importance and value of research in nursing. (Study of this topic enhances the socialization process.)
5. Professional ethics. (This would include the rights of subjects as well as the rights of professional workers.)

At a more concrete level, Fleming would expect students to (1) form a definition of research, (2) differentiate between research and problem solving, (3) differentiate between nursing research and research in nursing, (4) describe the steps of research, (5) write abstracts of research, (6) value research in nursing, and (7) understand the ethics of research.

Murdaugh, Kramer, and Schmalenberg (1981) report the findings of a survey of the NLN-accredited schools of nursing that focused on the teaching of nursing research. Of the 41 schools supplying data, none required a thesis at the baccalaureate level, although at three schools students could elect to write a thesis. Twelve (29 percent) of the programs required students to complete a research project. The authors conclude that baccalaureate programs emphasize intelligent consumership of research.

Castles (1984) argues for a required research course at the baccalaureate level, with the major objective of the course being to enable the student to view research critically. The content would include the steps of the research process, the application of that information in the critical review of research reports, and exposure to researchers and research. The focus is research utilization or application to practice.

Kim (1984) offers a conceptual typology for determining behavioral outcomes related to research teaching at the undergraduate level. The typology includes three perspectives: general, formal, and utilitarian. The general perspective encompasses the knowledge, skills, and attitudes needed for development of the underlying qualities essential for using scientific approaches to problem solving. The formal perspective encompasses the knowledge, skills, and attitudes needed in the research process and the methods essential for conducting research. The utilitarian perspective encompasses the knowledge, skills, and attitudes needed for effective utilization of research findings and competence as a consumer of research. The behavioral outcomes relevant to each perspective are listed in Table 1.

Overfield and Duffy (1984) review the research literature on teaching research to undergraduate nursing students. They propose that the subject matter for research courses should be determined according to the positions students are expected to be eligible to fill on gradu-

Table 1
Behavioral Outcomes for Three Perspectives on Research Teaching in Undergraduate Nursing Curricula*

Perspective	Behavioral Outcomes
General	1. Demonstrate intellectual curiosity. 2. Differentiate types of knowledge. 3. Differentiate methodologies of knowledge generation. 4. Use inductive and deductive approaches for problem solving and analysis of ideas.
Formal	1. Identify the major elements of research process and the interrelationships among the elements. 2. Define and use basic terminology in research. 3. Identify simple problems for research. 4. Select and critically review literature. 5. Identify basic qualitative and quantitative approaches to data analysis. 6. Identify implications of nursing practice for nursing research. 7. Use nursing practice as a means of data gathering for refining and extending nursing practice.
Utilitarian	1. Read research reports and understand overall meanings of reports. 2. Criticize research findings with respect to the major elements of research process, meaning, appropriateness, and value. 3. Identify potential applications of research findings in nursing practice.

*From the University of Rhode Island College of Nursing Curriculum Workshop, January 1979.

ation or capable of achieving shortly thereafter. On this basis, they propose that students be taught to be readers and users of research.

Reed (1985) envisions undergraduate students learning about the research process by developing their own small group research proposal; however, she adds that the content should include theory and metatheory.

Heaney and Barger-Lux (1986) describe the undergraduate research course at Creighton University's School of Nursing, the goal of which is to teach students to read research critically and to be professional consumers of research. They do not consider knowing how to do research to be part of beginning professional nursing practice. The course has three major elements: problem solving in a context of variability, critical reading of the research literature, and ethical dimensions of human investigation.

Duffy's (1986) review of the literature comes to three conclusions:

1. Research books used as course texts in undergraduate research courses are slowly being revised to reflect the growing trend to prepare students to be knowledgeable consumers of research rather than primarily doers of research.
2. Many authors believe that undergraduate research course content should include the nature of theory and the role it plays in nursing research; the elements of the research process; application of the research process to critical appraisal and use of research; the nature of research and the role that research plays in nursing; and the rights of research participants and of researchers.
3. The role of statistics and computer science in relation to research is undetermined.

THE WHEN OF TEACHING RESEARCH

Ludeman (1979) argues that the curriculum should reflect the philosophy of the school and its faculty. If nursing is seen as a science, research should be taught early in the curriculum as separate courses and be integrated into all upper division courses. If the faculty views nursing as a care giving, service oriented discipline, research would be taught less and later. At Montana State University, nursing research is taught at the junior level and at least one research objective is incorporated in all of the clinical courses. It has been helpful to have juniors work with more experienced RN students on research projects.

Thiel (1984) reports the findings of a longitudinal comparative study undertaken to assess the consequences of having nursing students at the University of Idaho take the nursing research class in the second year of the baccalaureate program. The study, conducted over a three-year period, showed that early placement of the course in the program increased the students' application of research (only 19 percent of those who took the course as seniors worked on a project, whereas 65 percent of those who took the course as sophomores did). Sophomores tended to select more scholarly reference sources: 50 percent used *Nursing Research*, whereas only 37 percent of the juniors did. Sophomores and juniors reported more enthusiasm about research than seniors did. After taking the course, 87 percent of the juniors, 88 percent of the sophomores, and 67 percent of the seniors were applying research to their clinical practice.

THE HOW OF TEACHING RESEARCH

I present the following recommendations on strategies for teaching research in chronological order. Many of the reports from which the recommendations are taken are descriptions of individual projects of limited generalizability. Nonetheless, they provide valuable information on teaching research at the undergraduate level.

Marriner (1980) describes teaching a required research course to more than 100 students every week. Besides having to take two examinations, students were required to complete a group research proposal and group written and oral critiques of a published nursing research study. The groups were small, which kept the class to a manageable size. The course evaluation revealed that students found the clear, informative syllabus useful, liked the examples used in lectures, felt that writing a research proposal forced them to put principles into practice, learned from doing a critique, and even learned from other group members. Students were enthusiastic about guest speakers, and many of them demonstrated an improved attitude toward research in the second half of the term.

Wilson (1982) outlines four themes that have helped her to convert "reluctant students to aspiring nurse scientists." The first theme is *criticality*, the objective being to enhance the spirit of inquiry and encourage students to approach experiences with a curious, analytic mind. She devoted time to teaching active reading skills and working on critical and reflective thinking and problem solving. The second theme is *communality*, i.e., exposing students to guest lecturers, workshops, conferences, and faculty role modeling and mentorship. The third theme is *continuity*, i.e., demonstrating that research is a part of nursing, linking research to practice, encouraging students to see the connection between their own scholarly work and clinical practice, and collaborating with other faculty so that research is integrated into other nursing courses. The fourth theme is the *research climate*, i.e., ensuring that faculty is involved in research, that there is good access to resources and an adequate library, and that teachers are enthusiastic.

Goshman (1983) describes a teaching strategy that involved students in faculty research. Selected senior level students taking a family/child nursing course at Montana State University were given the opportunity to work with a faculty member in a research project. The study took two and a half years to complete. At the end of each quarter, students reported on progress made in some aspect of this ongoing study. Goshman believes baccalaureate students gained considerable understanding of the value of research from their participation in this project.

Shelley (1983) presents an instructor-directed research (IDIR) model as one approach to resolving some of the problems encountered in teaching research. In this model, "instructors design, conceptualize, integrate with existing knowledge and ongoing research and present for class execution an IDIR project which the instructor oversees from beginning to end" (p. 302). Students learn by doing; for instance, they learn to critique by reading instructor-selected journal articles. In this way, they learn research methods and get high quality experience while their instructors enjoy a better chance of surviving the "publish or perish" trap. Research and teaching are integrated; beginning students can implement research, read significant research, and possibly participate in generating new knowledge. The entire process is designed and planned by the instructor, who gets sole credit for publication, though teams of students write final reports based on their own analysis of class-pooled data.

Johnson (1984) notes in her literature review that the articles published on strategies for teaching research do not include teaching statistics in research classes. At the University of Texas, students are introduced to research at the senior level. A period of 14 hours is devoted to the research process, with one hour devoted to statistical analysis. Deeming this inadequate, the author developed a strategy for teaching research by integrating statistics and research concepts. She uses data generated from a pretest on basic procedures and concepts in statistics. These data are incorporated into class discussions as each step of the research process is covered. This strategy has lessened stress, made the class more meaningful, and changed the basic format of the class from lecture to discussion.

Sweeney (1984) describes the use of a poster session teaching strategy to teach students to analyze, condense, and visually communicate the results of nursing research studies. During the semester, students worked on preparing a poster session, using a nursing research-based study of their choice. The instructor gave directions during the first class session, taking pains to encourage creativity. The posters were judged by other faculty, and the author concluded that the session "seemed to operationalize, integrate and synthesize the learning experience" (p. 137). Besides being exposed to a variety of research projects and presentations, students were able to view others' work.

Given nursing educators' increasing focus on developing positive research attitudes with a process orientation, rather than on teaching factual information on research techniques, Sakalys (1985) proposes developmentally oriented questioning as a process-oriented strategy for teaching the intellectual skills and attitudes of inquiry basic to the research role. She discusses the development of decision-making and problem-solving capabilities by describing theories of levels of development and reasoning abilities, then goes on to address "developmental instruction." She suggests that nursing educators, if they wish to promote a "research attitude," should make questioning about hypothetical dilemmas (i.e., the Socratic method) a part of teaching. The level of questioning should be determined by the student's developmental level. These teaching strategies will challenge and stimulate students to improve their cognitive and critical abilities.

Bzdek and Ganong (1986) describe a teaching methodology designed to introduce the steps of the research process to undergraduate students. This approach included participation in a study designed and carried out by the class. The project required three class sessions, and data were collected during spring break. The students compared the image of nurses held by Missourians to the damaging television stereotypes identified by Kalisch, Kalisch, and Scobey (1983). The 57 students were thus introduced to research concepts in the context of a real project rather than in the context of a textbook list.

Dean (1986) describes a strategy for teaching research by participant observation. The nursing instructor, head nurse, and staff nurse collaborated on an 18-month study aimed at determining the effect of an intervention designed to facilitate parent-infant bonding. Students were second-semester juniors in a baccalaureate program whose clinical experience was in the maternity unit. At the University of Connecticut, where this study was done, formal research content is taught in the first semester of the senior year. Considerable enthusiasm and interest were aroused in the students as they observed the progression of the research project.

Harris (1986) describes how she developed computer-assisted instruction (CAI) lessons for a nursing research course. Students who took her class on validity and reliability applied their knowledge as well as those who took other research classes in conventional classrooms.

Hastings-Tolsma and Brockopp (1986) discuss neurolinguistic programming (NLP) as a way of stimulating interest in research among nursing students. According to the literature, successful teaching of research skills requires an experienced teacher, small group discussions, "doable" activities, and involvement of students in some or all aspects of the research process. The NLP model is based on the relationship between learning and an individual's sensory organization; most education is based on visual and auditory-verbal skills. The authors urge that educators vary their approaches and make greater use of the kinesthetic modes, (emotion, enthusiasm, physical activity, and other sensory strategies).

Powers and Smith (1986) describe having senior nursing students conduct quality assurance studies in the clinical setting as part of a research course. The hospital quality assurance coordinators submit suggestions for studies they would like done on current patient care problems. Not only does this program involve collaboration between nursing practice and education, it also fosters development of problem-solving skills and encourages students to establish relationships with staff nurses, which will allow them to be assimilated more quickly and easily into the hospital work force.

Brand (1987) describes options for research teaching. At the University of Minnesota, all baccalaureate nursing students are required to take an introductory research course in their junior year, which must follow at least two clinical nursing courses. In that course, research process and terminology are taught with a focus on helping students to become skilled consumers of research. In their senior year, students take a one-credit course in which they can either work with a preceptor on ongoing research or design and execute a project alone. Usually one to six students work with each of approximately 15 preceptors per quarter. Students formulate a research question within the preceptor's study, then work independently, write a report, and give an oral presentation at the end of the quarter. A dynamic research environment in which willing preceptors work on a variety of studies is important, and it is helpful to have graduate programs present at the school.

Harrison, Hubbard, and Lane (1987) report a strategy for promoting research application among baccalaureate nursing students through confirmation of qualitative research. At the end of the senior year, students participate in an eight-week clinical practicum, working 40 hours a week with a registered nurse preceptor. One of the objectives is to teach students to utilize inquiry methodology and incorporate relevant research findings into practice. The authors describe how two students working in neonatal intensive care units (NICUs) attempted to confirm the findings of a qualitative study on how nurses in an NICU "created meaning" and dealt with the stress of their jobs. The students observed how nurses in their units functioned and reported on it.

Thiel (1987) describes a teaching strategy in which students taste two types of cookies and then hold a discussion comparing the two. The author found it to be a painless and creative way of introducing students to the research process.

Are these the solutions to the difficulties nursing has encountered in teaching research to undergraduate students? If we incorporate all these recommendations into our teaching, will entry-level practitioners begin to incorporate research into their practice more systematically? Will the problems Katefian (1975) identified in her study of research utilization be solved? I think not, because there remains a fundamental question that these approaches do not fully address.

RELATIONSHIP BETWEEN THEORY, PRACTICE, AND RESEARCH

In my view, the most critical issue in the teaching of research is the underlying conception of the relationship between theory, practice, and research. The traditional view of this relationship is well described by Fawcett (1980):

> The only way to generate, refine, or enlarge the knowledge needed by nursing is through scientific research. Therefore, it is incumbent upon nurses to conduct investigations of nursing phenomena. However, unless this research is guided by theory and unless the theory is tested through research, both are in danger of being isolated and therefore trivial enterprises. Moreover, since the ultimate aim of all nursing theory and research is to improve the quality of client care, theory and research must have some bearing on nursing practice.

Figure 1 is a simple schematic representation of the traditional model of the relationships between theory, practice, and research. This model has five important identifying characteristics. First, the primary responsibility for developing the knowledge base is ascribed to the scientist. Second, the primary source of knowledge is external to the practitioner-client setting. Third, the practitioner is expected to value and use the scientist-generated knowledge base in practice. Fourth, the practitioner is a conduit for knowledge to be used in the real world. Fifth, the client is not a part of the process of generating knowledge.

Schon (1983) labels the traditional model of the relationship between knowledge (theory and research) and practice "technical rationality" and links it to positivism. He offers three descriptors of the model of technical rationality:

Figure 1
Traditional Model of the Relationship Between Theory, Practice and Research in Nursing

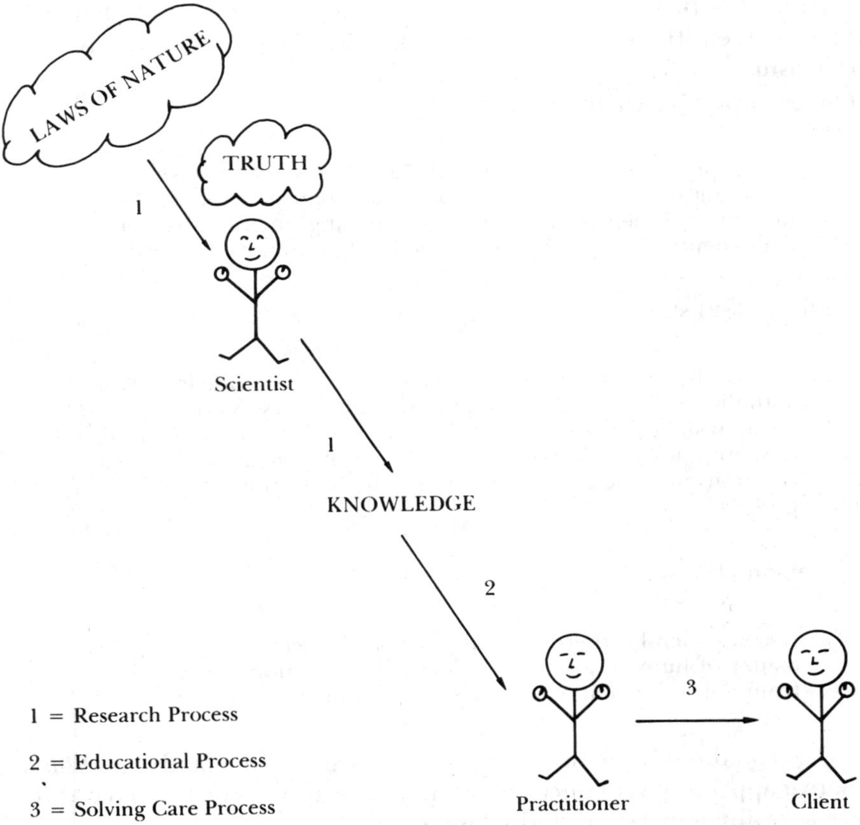

Professional activity consists in instrumental problem solving made rigorous by the application of scientific theory and technique.

The systematic knowledge base of a profession is thought to have four essential properties. It is specialized, firmly founded, scientific, and *standardized.*

If every professional problem were in all respects unique, solutions would be at best accidental, and therefore having nothing to do with expert knowledge. What we are suggesting, on the con-

> trary, is that there must be sufficient uniformities in problems and in devices for solving them to qualify the solvers as professionals. . . . *professionals apply very general principles, standardized knowledge, to concrete problems*. . . .

Although this paradigm has strong advocates and underlies many of our scientific, educational, and practice activities, it is also under criticism.

For example, Newman (1982) remarks:

> The prevailing methodology of nursing research is grounded in the scientific method, which is based on context stripping. Yet the human experience—the focus of nursing inquiry—is context-dependent; i.e., it can be understood only within its own text.

Ellis (1982) states:

> It is also my thesis that the generation of knowledge involves both discovery and validation and that the processes are related but distinguishable phases that differ considerably. Few would argue this, but it is common among those who functionally seem to equate research and science to focus only on the testing and validation process.

Watson (1983) adds:

> Consequently, there is a disjunction between nursing's subject matter of human care and the methodologies nurses have adopted from the traditional natural sciences and medicine.

One could easily go on to consider the issues of qualitative and quantitative approaches, deductive and inductive approaches, borrowed theory and nursing theory, and so forth.

I believe that what we need is not just a revised traditional model but a new model that links theory, practice and research by first focusing on practice and then letting the nature of nursing itself determine the nature of our knowledge and the methods for developing it. Consequently, it is appropriate for us to reflect on the future of health care rather than on the past. It is time to be critical of the so-called rules of science, which have not been changed for a half-century.

Fries (1985) summarizes the major changes in health conditions and medical expenditures as follows:

- 1900s — Era of acute infectious disease, with over 70 percent of the illness burden due to such conditions
- Currently — Illness burden shifted to chronic, non-infectious illnesses, such as atherosclerosis, cancer, diabetes, emphysema, and arthritis
- Emerging — Major health problems related to the aging of the population rather than specific illnesses and to the stress of a rapidly changing world, including its infrastructures.

He supports a view of natural evolution that is linked with scientific advances and argues that the medical model that grew out of the acute infectious disease era is partially inadequate for chronic, non-infectious diseases and totally inadequate for aging and stress- or lifestyle-related health problems.

A new model of the relationship between theory, practice, and research (Figure 2) would then begin by depicting the provider-client component as an interaction and placing it in a specific context. It would show both practitioners and researchers reflecting on practice as a source of knowledge and applying methods of disciplined inquiry to that practice arena. Knowledge generated through the inquiry of both practitioners and researchers would be actively discussed and evaluated before it was considered knowledge for the discipline.

Basic to this paradigm are five assumptions: First, the care process is designed to help people to help themselves. Second, the life of knowledge is short—four years or less. Third, knowledge is context-specific, because of its short lifespan and the complexity of the problems addressed. Fourth, improving the quality of life is the goal of science; science will be both pragmatic and humanitarian. Fifth, generating knowledge is an interactive, iterative process. The goal of research is to generate knowledge that people can use to design and execute their actions in their daily relationships at all levels.

Does a paradigm such as this address the objections raised to the traditional model of science? Obviously, the model presented in Figure 2 is only a first step toward reconceptualizing the traditional paradigm. I believe, however, that it represents a major departure from tradition, one that addresses both criticisms of the current situation and predictions for the future.

One set of guidelines that reflects a new concept of research utilization was developed by Tanner (1987). A modification of this set of guidelines is the basis for a forthcoming research text for undergraduate students to be published by the NLN.

Figure 2
New Model of the Relationship Between Theory, Practice, and Research in Nursing

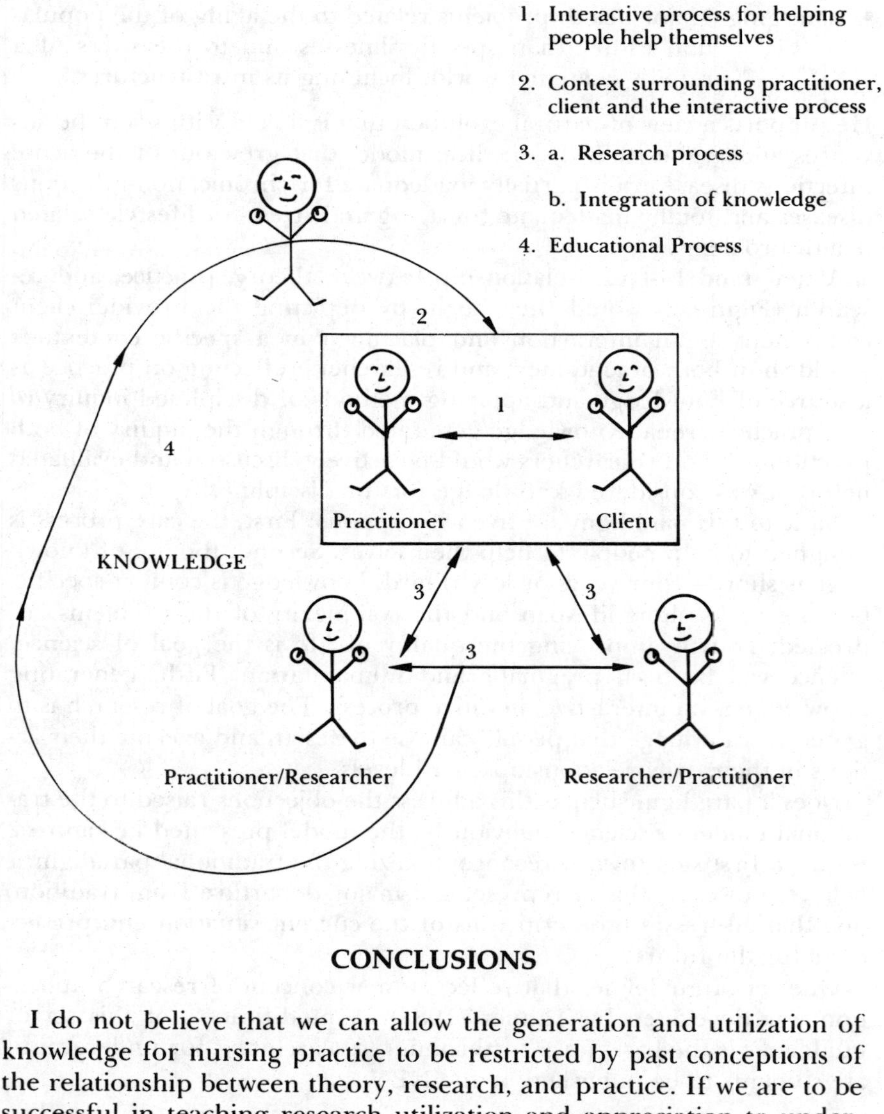

CONCLUSIONS

I do not believe that we can allow the generation and utilization of knowledge for nursing practice to be restricted by past conceptions of the relationship between theory, research, and practice. If we are to be successful in teaching research utilization and appreciation to undergraduate students, our conception of the relationship between research and practice must reflect the present and the future, not the past. A real curriculum revolution must include increased attention to underlying conceptions, not just to new methods for teaching the same old ideas. Our ability to question, to probe, and to inquire is inseparable from who and what we are. In this act of being, nothing is sacred, not even the paradigm from which we operate.

REFERENCES

Brand, K. P. (1987). Options for clinical nursing research experiences. *Nurse Educator, 12*(2), 35–39.

Burkhalter, P. K., & Kim, H. T. (1976). The Honors Program approach to undergraduate research in nursing. *Journal of Nursing Education, 15*(1): 46–51.

Bzdek, V. M. & Ganong, L. H. (1986). Teaching the research process through participatory learning. *Nursing Educator, 11*(6), 24–28

Castles, M. R. (1984). Teaching research methods in schools of nursing. *Journal of Nursing Education, 23*(3), 120–121.

Dean, P. G. (1986). Strategies for teaching nursing research: Participant observation. *Western Journal of Nursing Research, 8*(3), 278–282.

Downs, F. S. (1980, January/February). Teaching nursing research: Strategies. *Nurse Educator*, pp. 27–29.

Duffy, M. E. (1986). Nursing research at the baccalaureate level. *Nursing & Health Care*, 7(6), 293–295.

Duffy, M. E. (1987). The research process in baccalaureate nursing education: A ten-year review. *Image: Journal of Nursing Scholarship, 19*(2), 87–91.

Ellis, R. (1982). Editorial. *Advances in Nursing Science, 4*(4), x–xi.

Fawcett, J. (1980, June). A declaration of nursing independence: The relation of theory and research to nursing practice. *The Journal of Nursing Administration*, 36–39.

Fleming, J. (1980). Teaching nursing research: Content. *Nurse Educator, 5*(1), 24–26.

Fries, J. F. (1985, July). *The future of disease and treatment: Changing health conditions, changing behaviors, and new medical technology.* Paper presented at "Nursing in the 21st Century," a conference of the American Association of Colleges of Nursing and the American Organization of Nurse Executives, Aspen, CO.

Goshman, B. (1983). Strategies for teaching nursing research: Involving students in faculty research. *Western Journal of Nursing Research, 5*(3), 250–253.

Harris, S. L. (1986). Development of computer-assisted instruction lessons for teaching nursing research. *Computer Nursing, 4*(4), 140–182.

Harrison, L. L., Hubbard, L., & Lane, J. (1987). Confirmation of qualitative research findings in the clinical setting: A strategy to promote research application among baccalaureate nursing students. *Journal of Nursing Education, 26*(5), 208–210.

Hastings-Tolsma, J. T., & Brockopp, D. Y. (1986). Stimulating research: A sensory model. *Western Journal of Nursing Research, 8*(2), 197–205.

Heaney, R. P., & Barger-Lux, M. J. (1986). Priming students to read research critically. *Nursing & Health Care, 7*(8): 420–424.

Johnson, J. M. (1984). Strategies for teaching nursing research: Strategies for including statistical concepts in a course in research methodology for baccalaureate nursing students. *Western Journal of Nursing Research, 6*(2), 259–264.

Kalisch, P. A., Kalisch, B. J., & Scobey, M. (1983). *Images of nurses on television.* New York: Springer Publishing Company.

Katefian, S. (1975). Application of selected nursing research findings into nursing practice. *Nursing Research, 24*(2), 89–92.

Kim, H. S. (1984). Critical contents of research process for an undergraduate nursing curriculum. *Journal of Nursing Education, 23*(2), 70–72.

Ludeman, R. (1979). Strategies for teaching nursing research: Placement of research content in the undergraduate curriculum. *Western Journal of Nursing Research, 1*(3), 260–263.

Marriner, A. (1980). Strategies for teaching nursing research: Research preparation in baccalaureate nursing education. *Western Journal of Nursing Research, 2*(2), 539–542.

Murdaugh, C., Kramer, M., & Schmalenberg, C. E. (1981). The teaching of nursing research: A survey report. *Nurse Educator, 6*(1), 28–35.

Newman, Margaret. (1982). Editorial. *Advances in Nursing Science, 5*(2), x–xi.

Overfield, T., & Duffy, M. E. (1984). Research on teaching research in the baccalaureate nursing curriculum. *Journal of Advanced Nursing, 9*, 189–196.

Powers, B. A., & Smith, T. C. (1986). An approach to undergraduate student investigations in clinical settings. *Image: Journal of Nursing Scholarship, 18*(1), 15–17.

Reed, P. G. (1985). Strategies for teaching research: Theory and metatheory in an undergraduate research course. *Western Journal of Nursing Research, 7*(4), 482–485.

Sakalys, J. A. (1985). Strategies for teaching nursing research: Developing a research attitude through questioning. *Western Journal of Nursing Research, 7*(2), 254–260.

Schon, D. (1983). *The reflective practitioner.* New York: Basic Books.

Shelley, S. I. (1983). The IDIR model for faculty research with students. *Western Journal of Nursing Research, 5*(4), 301–312.

Sweeney, S. S. (1984). Strategies for teaching nursing research: Poster sessions for undergraduate students: A useful tool for learning and communicating nursing research. *Western Journal of Nursing Research, 6*(1), 135–138.

Tanner, C. A. (1987, July). Evaluating research for use in practice: Guidelines for the clinician. *Heart & Lung, 16*(4): 424–431.

Thiel, C. A. (1987). The cookie experiment: A creative teaching strategy. *Nurse Educator, 12*(3), 8–20.

Thiel, J. (1984). Strategies for teaching nursing research: Placement of research: Does it make a difference? *Western Journal of Nursing Research, 6*(3), 356–358.

Watson, J. (1983, October). Unpublished keynote presentation to Faculty, School of Nursing, University of Colorado, Boulder, CO.

Wilson, H. S. (1982). Teaching research in nursing: Issues and strategies. *Western Journal of Nursing Research, 4*(4), 365–377.